Living Healthy

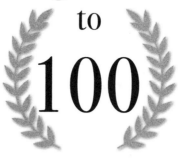

to

100

A Wellness Program
for Seniors

M.B. Seretean

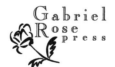

Gabriel
Rose
press

Living Healthy to 100
A Wellness Program for Seniors

Author: M.B. Seretean

Publication Date: Autumn 2005

Paperback edition price: $17.95 USA / $4.95 shipping
$19.95 Canada / $6.95 shipping

Finished size: 5 3/8 x 8 3/8
Number of pages: 328
Publisher: Gabriel Rose Press, Inc.

Seretean, M.B., 1924
Living Healthy to 100
Self Help Guide
Includes Resources

Library of Congress Control Number: 2005931283

ISBN 0-9649301-4-5
978-0-9649301-4-8

Living Healthy to 100 is intended as a guide to living a healthier lifestyle for those over 55 and should be used as a supplement to conventional medical care, not a replacement. Readers, especially those facing medical challenges, should consult a physician before making lifestyle changes discussed in this book.

TABLE OF CONTENTS

PREFACE

For Bud Seretean, the awakening came suddenly and unexpectedly.

A self-made businessman who built one of the nation's most successful carpet manufacturing firms from scratch, Seretean was in his mid-50s and enjoying what he believed was reasonably good health in 1979 when he stumbled upon the Pritikin Longevity Center in Downington, Pa.

There he discovered that, despite letters from top physicians giving him a clean bill of health, he wasn't nearly as healthy as he believed. Among the first tasks at hand were to bring his overall cholesterol down from 270 and reduce his blood pressure, primarily through diet and exercise.

Seretean's two-week stay at the Pritikin center served as the genesis for a complete change in the way he lived. For most of his first five-and-a-half decades, Seretean had been living a lifestyle that put him on an almost certain collision course with serious illness. But, using what he learned at Pritikin as a foundation, Seretean soon began a journey that has led him to a much healthier and fuller life. His goal is to be photographed working out in a gym on his 100th birthday.

For more than a quarter of a century, Seretean has dedicated himself to learning as much as he can about living a healthy lifestyle. Now in his 80s, he continues on a rigorous exercise and healthy eating regimen every day and lives an active lifestyle that would make many in their 50s and 60s envious. He abides by the philosophy that aging is a treatable condition and that now is the time to stop the clock. He is living proof that a healthy lifestyle can have an impact on the aging process.

Seretean also believes all individuals need to take responsibility for their own health. He believes all men and women, especially those over 55, can add years to their lives through effective and simple lifestyle changes, primarily in the areas of diet and exercise.

Helping others discover the health secrets he has found has been a driving passion for Seretean, who founded the Seretean Wellness Center on the campus of Oklahoma State University, the first of its kind on a university campus, and the M.B. Seretean Health Promotion Center at Emory University.

PREFACE

In writing this book, Seretean hopes to share with the growing number of seniors information he collected that will lead to a healthier and happier life during the later years – which he believes should be the "golden" years instead of the "olden" or sick years.

Seretean is often called upon to speak on diet, exercise and a healthier lifestyle. He has attended a number of intensive wellness programs and has followed the philosophies of Nathan Pritikin, Dr. Dean Ornish and Dr. Walter Willett of Harvard University. As he has done in his presentations, Seretean has focused this book on seven key topics, which will each make up a section.

Those topics include:
- Nutrition
- Exercise
- Maintaining a Healthy Weight
- Stress Control
- Alcohol, Tobacco and Drugs – Control of Substance Abuse
- Accident, Injury, and Illness Prevention
- The Value of a Healthy Mind and Attitude

As you read through these pages, you'll see they are a compilation of Seretean's knowledge and personal experiences designed to help enrich the lives of readers. By following in Seretean's footsteps, there is a good chance readers may live longer and feel and look better every day of the rest of their lives.

AUTHOR'S NOTE

As you go through this book, you will see that the type is easy to read, the chapters often are short and the concepts are easy to understand. My goal in writing this book has always been to help people – especially those over 55 – find a way to live a healthier lifestyle, and I felt the best way to do that was to follow the KIS method – Keep It Simple. Since I am not a doctor, I avoided complicated explanations most of us wouldn't understand. Instead, my focus is to share with you some of the knowledge that works for me and that I have discovered through reading and research during the last 25 years.

Throughout the book, you will find color photos that will help illustrate some of the exercises I describe and you'll also find color photos and recipes of some of the healthy meals you can prepare without straying from a healthy lifestyle. Healthy foods can and should be colorful.

This book was written with the hope that others will discover the benefits of living a healthy lifestyle and will make some changes that will lead to a better quality of life now and for years to come. If one person's life is changed for the better, then all of the work that went into this effort will have been worthwhile. Remember, it is never too late to start.

Hoping that many of you will live to celebrate your 100th birthday – in good health.

M.B. "Bud" Seretean

ACKNOWLEDGMENTS

Writing a book is an ambitious endeavor, and I could not have done it without the help and support of dozens of people. Over the years, I have been inspired and motivated by many, including Nathan Pritikin, Dr. Dean Ornish and Dr. Walter Willett. I have also been inspired by people like Jack LaLanne, who is living proof that a healthy lifestyle can make for a longer and better life.

This book could not have been written without the help of Rich Pollack and Carol Csomay of Pollack Communications in Delray Beach, Florida, who worked with me to write, edit and rewrite the words on every page. My sincerest thanks also goes out to Tom Baggot, an executive chef and personal trainer, who has worked with me for several years and who provided the recipes listed in the back of this book that are served frequently in my home. Helping to make this book easy to read were my longtime friend and fellow author, Anne Benham, and my daughter, Tracy Seretean, an Academy Award-winning film producer. In addition, my appreciation goes out to Richard Sheremeta of AlpenGlow Productions for his photography. I also want to express my gratitude to Dr. Mac McCrory and the entire staff at the Seretean Wellness Center for their help in providing support and scientific information.

Finally, I want to thank all of those who have heard me speak on this topic and whose enthusiasm led me to see the value a book such as this can have in improving people's lives.

WHY READ THIS BOOK?

As you thumb through the pages of this book, you may start to notice it's a little different than most other books focused on healthy lifestyles.

Many of those books are written by either doctors or nutritionists. I am neither.

Others are written by celebrities who lend their names to a diet or endorse a shake that's supposed to help you slim down, so they and their wallets can get fat – literally and figuratively. I'm frankly not interested in financial gains from this project; in fact, all of the proceeds from this book will go to supporting research about healthy lifestyles.

Still other books are written by well-educated and well-meaning doctors who can help you lose weight through dieting but who don't address other key issues that are vital to maintaining a healthy lifestyle.

If all you're looking for is another weight-loss program, then this book is not for you. However, if you're looking for a healthy lifestyle plan that incorporates different facets of living well, this book should offer many worthwhile ideas.

This book is simply a collection of insights about healthy living from a man who has been studying the subject – and living it – for two-and-a-half decades. And it is written with people over 55 years old in mind.

Unlike some of the authors in this field, I practice what I preach. I have made it to 80 by doing most of the right things health-wise for the last 25 years. Now I am committed to trying harder and being somewhat smarter to make it through the next 20 years.

What I've tried to do in this book is give you an idea of what has been and still is working for me. My hope is that by sharing this story, I will help others see the benefits and realize it's never too late to start eating better, exercising more and stressing out less.

Throughout this book, I write about my experiences. In the section on stress, for example, you'll see I lived a very stressful life for many years but through education and practice, I figured out how best to keep stress from damaging my health.

You'll see I've learned it's not so bad to park a little farther from the store and walk a little, and that dancing can be exercise and fun at the same time. And you'll find that good food doesn't have to taste bad and that a commitment to a healthy lifestyle is far from a vow of deprivation.

This book also tells you about the foods I eat and my philosophy on nutrition as well as the exercises I do to keep body fat down and my spirits up.

Of course, *Living Healthy to 100* doesn't just tell you what I've done, but also covers all I've learned from being a student, a teacher and a collector of knowledge from many sources on this subject.

Recipes that are relatively easy to prepare are included, as well as step-by-step instructions through the preparation process. But I'll also take you shopping, tell you what to look for when you're walking down the aisles of the local supermarket and even point out aisles to avoid that are potential landmines for someone trying to maintain a healthy diet.

My goal, of course, is not to browbeat you or frighten you into a lifestyle that may or may not be right for you. Instead, the objective is to educate you about what has worked for me and others and show you how it can work for you.

You'll see that unlike what you find in diet books or some other healthy lifestyle books, you aren't presented with an all-or-nothing equation. Instead, you are offered opportunities to start at a level that's right for you and then work your way up to a place where you're comfortable.

Just because I exercise for 50 minutes every day, does that mean you should, too? Of course not. Realizing that most of our readers will be over 55, I offer you exercise advice that gives you the option to do as much as you physically can and then helps you build up to higher levels.

In addition to telling you what exercises have worked best for me, there are also instructions, in specific detail, about how to go about doing them. And photos have been included as well, illustrating everything from stretches to weight-training exercises.

While some books may delve deeply into why you should walk every day, this book will tell you more about how to get the most out of your walk.

And while other books may tell you how to lose weight, the goal here is to tell you how to avoid putting it on in the first place.

As I mentioned earlier, this book is not a weight-loss book. Instead, it is a lifestyle book based on what I've learned from attending programs at the Pritikin Longevity Center and from health seminars conducted

WHY READ THIS BOOK?

by Dr. Dean Ornish, in addition to what I've read and studied over the years. It is centered around the philosophy that diets low in unhealthy fats, complemented by lots of fruits, vegetables, whole grains and healthy fats – along with regular exercise – can help you live longer and healthier.

You'll find there are certain diets that are better than others, and I'll share that with you in the book's weight control section. I'll also share some dos and don'ts about weight loss with you.

That brings me to one important difference between this book and others you'll find on the market. My goal has always been to make this book as easy to read as possible. So there are lots of photos and illustrations and the chapters have been deliberately kept relatively short whenever possible. And most of the sections end with a dos and don'ts list.

That said, it seems only fitting to end this segment with a short dos and don'ts list about this book.

- Don't buy this book if you just want to lose weight.
- Read this book if you want to learn about a healthy lifestyle that has worked for me.
- Read this book if you want to learn the specifics of living a healthy lifestyle.
- Don't expect this book to help you reverse the effects of years of an unhealthy lifestyle overnight. It contains no magic bullet.
- Read this book if you believe it's never too late to start living better.
- Read this book if you're really committed to making a healthier lifestyle change.
- Read this book if you want to be a positive role model for your children, grandchildren and friends.
- Read this book if you want to live to 100 and be as healthy as you can during those years.

MY GURUS

Nathan Pritikin, Dr. Dean Ornish and Dr. Walter Willett are the three individuals whose expertise has provided me with most of the knowledge to lead a healthy lifestyle.

Nathan Pritikin

Nathan Pritikin was a pioneer in developing the concept that there is a relationship between health, diet, exercise and longevity. He was not a doctor but a man who developed heart disease and sought ways to cure it without surgery. As a result of studies over a long period that he made of healthy populations and their eating and lifestyle habits, he eliminated his heart problem and founded the Pritikin Longevity Center and the Institute for Healthy Aging. It was my first visit to a Pritikin Longevity Center that made me examine my own lifestyle and turned my unhealthy life around. It introduced me to a new concept of how to live.

While my blood pressure and cholesterol levels dropped during that first two-week program, I was the only one in the group who was relatively healthy. The others were people who were obese or suffering with advanced diabetes and/or heart disease. Those with heart problems were there as their last chance before having to face surgery. What is so amazing is that the health of all of these very unhealthy people improved dramatically in just two weeks.

Participants ate six times a day and engaged in quite a bit of exercise. We attended classes two or three hours a day to learn about major diseases, why they occur and how to treat them.

Pritikin co-authored the best-selling books *Live Longer Now* and *The Pritikin Program for Exercise and Health*. Later, he wrote *The Pritikin Permanent Weight-Loss Program*, geared toward people with moderate health problems such as slight hypertension but also toward other people who want to lose weight. All of the Pritikin diets are extremely low in fat, allowing only 10 percent to 15 percent total fat as part of the overall daily food intake.

Dr. Dean Ornish

Pritikin had most of the basics, but it was Dr. Dean Ornish who took Pritikin's work a step forward. He added his own knowledge and subjected all of it to extensive scientific research, which Pritikin didn't do. Dr. Ornish was also the first to recognize the importance of getting taste into the foods of a low-fat diet. The Pritikin diet was very bland. Dr. Ornish's food plan is similar to Pritikin's but more vegetarian and much tastier.

Dr. Ornish also introduced other elements such as yoga, meditation and weight training. He conducts interesting workshops, featuring physicians, chefs and nutritionists as speakers.

His initial research focused mainly on people with serious heart problems. He has conducted several scientific studies on heart patients utilizing a very low-fat, low-cholesterol diet and a healthy exercise regimen. Those studies revealed that this kind of program could improve the health of these patients. His book, *Dr. Dean Ornish's Program for Reversing Heart Disease*, was published in 1991. In it, he introduced the Opening Your Heart Program, which encompasses a very low-fat, almost vegetarian diet and safe exercise. It also includes a prevention diet, communication skills, various stress-reduction techniques, and information on how to stop smoking.

The book was a result of a 13-year study of heart patients that showed it's possible to lower cholesterol and high blood pressure, diminish or even eliminate chest pain, and help one become more energetic and lose weight while eating more food on a low-fat diet. His research also showed it is possible to reverse or even eliminate coronary blockages without surgery by a change in lifestyle.

I feel Dr. Ornish is far and away the most significant figure in America in the reversing and prevention of heart disease. He is also an advocate who took his findings to Congress and the White House. Most significantly, Dr. Ornish was able to get his program into a number of hospitals and persuade insurance companies to pay for it, in hopes it would eliminate the need for much more costly heart surgery. For people with this condition, I would definitely advocate Dr. Ornish's program, in conjunction with consultation with their physicians.

He exposed me to solid scientific research. I actually met the people in his research program when I was attending one of his seminars in

California. More recently, Dr. Ornish has been conducting research on prostate cancer and diet, showing that a very low-fat diet can lead to a reduction in size of the cancer or keep it from spreading. He is also looking into the relationship between diet and breast cancer.

Dr. Ornish's 1993 book *Eat More, Weigh Less* concentrates more on achieving a healthy weight and maintaining it, not only for people who may be ill, but also for others who want to lose weight and keep it off. Although the title may seem to suggest it is an ordinary diet book, it actually focuses mainly on making lifestyle changes that can help people become as healthy as possible. This still very low-fat, low-cholesterol, high-carbohydrate diet worked well when it was combined with exercise and stress reduction in a small but long-term study over five years.

Dr. Walter Willett

Reading Dr. Walter Willett's book, *Eat, Drink and Be Healthy*, introduced me to the reality of healthy fats. Dr. Willett's contention is that it's OK to have 30 percent or more fat in the diet as long as it is mainly healthy unsaturated fat. That would include monounsaturated fats and polyunsaturated fats such as omega-3.

Dr. Willett is a former chairman of the Department of Nutrition at the Harvard School of Public Health and the Frederick John Stare Professor of Epidemiology and Nutrition in those departments. He has been involved in a number of well-known studies showing that replacing saturated fat with unsaturated fat improves health. One of his other recommendations is that people replace some carbohydrates in their diets with healthy fats.

Dr. Willett has challenged many theories about food that have been taken for granted. One result is his version of a healthy food pyramid, which I believe is a great improvement over the USDA's food pyramid.

INTRODUCTION

What a great time to be alive!

It's a time many of us have waited for – these senior years, our golden years.

For decades, most of us focused on raising our children, building our careers and taking care of those everyday parts of life that often got in the way of our dreams. We talked about how someday we would go back to school, travel around the world, volunteer for something we really believe in or learn to play the piano. Somehow, though, we never got around to it.

Now those days are here. In most cases, our children are grown and have started their own lives. We have passed down the knowledge we learned in our careers to the next generation. Hopefully, we've put a few dollars aside so we can enjoy the remaining years.

We now have before us a blank canvas waiting to be filled with the colors from an endless palate. Yet without our health, those colors lack the vivid brightness that makes the painting complete.

There is so much still to do, and there are so many challenges lining our paths, so many adventures yet to embark upon that we may all need another 30 or 40 healthy years added onto our lives so we can experience it all.

I know I certainly do.

There are those who will say you are in the twilight years once you reach your 60s or 70s. If that's the case, I am hoping for a very long twilight.

As you read through the pages of this book, you'll see that my objective is to be a role model for all whose goal is "Living Healthy – to 100."

But for too many people, the thought of living to 100 is full of fright because they believe they will never be healthy enough to endure or enjoy the journey. There is a fear of being disabled, of suffering from the sicknesses that come with old age. Some fear that no matter what they do, genetics will win out and they will succumb to the same serious illnesses as their ancestors.

INTRODUCTION

The truth is, you can make a difference in the quality of your life and you can start today. If you do, chances are you'll feel better and look better for the rest of your life.

Even if you have medical problems or are genetically prone to a particular illness, any positive changes you make now will improve your chances of being able to combat any disease successfully or prevent it entirely.

So, this book is for people of any age, but primarily for those 55 and older, based on the idea that it is never too late to start living a healthy lifestyle. My goal is to help you, my readers, take control of your health and use that control to help you live a fuller life. If you don't take control of your health, no one else will. The responsibility lies with you.

My hope is that when you realize the benefits of healthy living, and realize it can be achieved, you'll see that the give-ups are minor compared with the gets.

Now, at this point you might be saying to yourself, "What qualifies him to give this advice?" Well, I think I'm a living example of what having a healthy lifestyle can do. I'm in my early 80s and I'm in better shape than I was a quarter of a century ago.

"OK," you say, "but you're not a doctor or a scientist."

It's true, I'm not. But for the past 25 years I've benefited from stays at three health promotion facilities and have read just about every health promotion book, magazine and newspaper article on health I could find. I've consulted with doctors and other health professionals at both my alma mater, Oklahoma State University, where I established the very first wellness center on a college campus, and at Emory University, where I provided the impetus for the M.B. Seretean Health Promotion Center.

I have also devoted the last 25 years to practicing what I am preaching.

I've committed myself to finding out all I could about the subject. I've been reading and studying and learning as much as I can, attending seminars, enrolling in additional programs and trying to live what I've learned – and I will be doing this the rest of my life.

After all, I have reason to learn about it more than any doctor does because I'm a member of this age group. My life is at stake.

I apologize to the reader for limiting the research to my personal healthy lifestyle experience. I wish I could provide you with some worthwhile scientific research on healthy living, involving many other individuals. But this book has taken one year to write and I didn't want to make it a five-year project – better to get it published now and hopefully benefit people sooner than later.

I'm often asked to speak about what I've learned. Now I want to share these insights with you, to share what I've discovered and what has worked for me, in the hopes that some of this information will work for you as well.

Throughout this book, you'll see that changes in your lifestyle, based in part on the theories of Nathan Pritikin, Dr. Dean Ornish and many others, can help you look better, feel better and most importantly, add healthy years to your life.

This book does not deliver a silver bullet. If you're looking for an easy answer, a pill, a workout contraption, perhaps a temporary diet or exercise program that you can adhere to for a few months, then you just might want to go back to the bookstore and get your money back.

What worked for me, and thousands of others like me, is a change in lifestyle centered on good nutrition, exercise, weight and stress control, positive thinking and just plain healthy living. It takes commitment and effort every day.

Because what good are these golden years if we are too sick or too feeble to enjoy them?

There is a quote I've read a hundred times that never ceases to amaze me with its brilliance, especially since it was written in 325 B.C. by Herophilus, the physician to Alexander the Great: "When health is absent, wisdom cannot reveal itself, art cannot become manifest, strength cannot fight and wealth becomes useless."

How true those words are today. You can't benefit from schooling or appreciate art when you are sick. You do not have the strength to do anything, and all the money in the world cannot buy back your health once you have lost it.

Have I had to make sacrifices? You bet. Are there days when I wake up and say, "I am too tired to work out"? Certainly. But what is clear to me is that the return I have received by changing my lifestyle and sticking with the program is many times greater than what I have had to give up.

I didn't always live this way. Like most Americans, I was doing a fine job of destroying my body for a good part of my life and not even knowing it. I had no clue that what I was really doing by leading my lifestyle – which included a high-fat diet, an insignificant amount of exercise and plenty of stress – was taking years off my life and destroying the joy in it as well.

I grew up the son of a grocer in New York City, and there was never a lack of food on our table. We thought we were eating healthfully by following the recommendations of the U.S. Department of Agriculture and trade association experts representing dairy farmers and cattle ranchers. Back then, I ate liver, hot dogs and other red meat, lots of cheese and butter, and I drank two quarts of milk a day. I also enjoyed numerous snacks and sweets. I really had no idea what a healthy diet was or how important it could be for sustaining my health.

My diet changed when I went into the military during World War II, but I simply went from one unhealthy diet to another.

As I made my way through college, getting both undergraduate and master's degrees, I was still on an unhealthy diet. I was getting somewhat more exercise but I was dealing with a great deal of stress, since I was four years behind others due to my military service and trying to make up the time.

As my career and then my business grew, I would grab lunches on the run and often skip meals to keep from disrupting a tight schedule. I still had a ton of stress.

In my late 40s I started thinking about my health. A close friend recommended I visit a world-famous clinic for a yearly, complete three-day checkup. Every year I would go there and leave with a letter from my doctor indicating I was in excellent health.

I never had reason for doubt until 1979.

My then-wife was a smoker who wanted to quit. She had tried just about everything available at that time – hypnosis, acupuncture, patches – and nothing worked. In her research, she had stumbled upon the Pritikin Longevity Center in Downington, Pa., and enrolled in its smoking cessation program. I went along to keep her company. The Pritikin center also offered two- and four-week programs for clients suffering from obesity, heart disease or diabetes.

When I arrived there, the Pritikin doctor asked if I was interested in enrolling in the program. I said I didn't think I needed to and showed him a letter indicating my healthy state. The doctor read the letter and started smiling as he pointed out to me some very poor numbers I was not familiar with.

My cholesterol, he told me, was 270, much too high, and my blood pressure was borderline hypertensive. He let me know that, in fact, I was a candidate for a heart attack if I didn't pursue a healthier diet and a much more aggressive exercise regimen and learn how to reduce the stress in my life. He also convinced me I was responsible for maintaining my health – that I shouldn't rely on doctors to prevent disease because most doctors were trained to treat disease and less prepared to teach you how to prevent it.

What a rude awakening! It was time for me to make a change.

I enrolled in the two-week course, which became a turning point in my life.

During my stay, I witnessed remarkable improvement in the health of the 55 people in our group. Daily and weekly checks of weight, blood work, blood pressure screenings and stress tests verified the progress. In my case, my overall cholesterol went down to 230 after two weeks, my blood pressure was 120 over 85 and my weight was down five pounds. All this was accomplished through a healthy low-fat diet and two hours of exercise a day. In addition, I went to classes taught by doctors three hours a day. The classes were on subjects such as the origins of diseases, the devastating effects of smoking and the reasons why the Pritikin program was so effective.

After leaving the Pritikin center, I decided to share what I had learned with others.

Since graduating from Oklahoma State (OSU) in 1949, I have become one of the most active alumni in the school's history, doing everything from teaching classes in a variety of subjects to hosting seminars that teach seniors how to prepare for job interviews.

Because of my Pritikin experience, I started investigating the state of health of the students and staff members on the campus. The head of the health promotion program at Oklahoma State asked me whether I would be interested in going to an annual wellness conference at the University of Wisconsin at Steven's Point. The conference, which I attended, included major health promotion experts from all over the country and this gave me the desire to do something special in wellness on the OSU campus.

INTRODUCTION

After learning about the limited wellness programs available at the school, I decided to make a gift that led Oklahoma State to build the first wellness center on any campus in the country. The 17 programs at the center, which opened in 1991 and has a full-time staff of 21, are aimed at students, faculty and staff and even people from the city of Stillwater, which is home to OSU.

Since its opening, I have been a guest lecturer and our programs have been so successful that we doubled our facilities and course offerings a few years ago. All freshmen are now given an opportunity to take a course in wellness taught by graduate students.

I have also been involved with Emory University in Atlanta and had served on the university's board of the School of Public Health. I noticed there was an opportunity for sharing information about wellness with the Centers for Disease Control and the American Cancer Society, both of which are headquartered on the campus, and the Emory University medical establishment. Consequently, I provided a gift to help build the Emory Seretean Center for Health Promotion.

I've also provided funding for research to Dr. Ornish – whose studies have documented that a healthy lifestyle can reverse the impact of heart disease and help in the treatment of prostate cancer – as well as to other researchers.

And I continue to read, listen and learn, because this is a subject in which the information is constantly changing and the science constantly improving.

On these pages, you will find discussions of seven areas key to a healthy lifestyle.

You may find that living 100 years is a realistic goal for you. It is a goal that will not only benefit you, but also the community as a whole. To quote the poet Robert Browning, "Your reach should exceed your grasp, for what are the Heavens for?" Shoot for 100 and the effort may get you to the 90s – that's not bad. Shoot for the 90s and you may only get to your 80s. Shoot for the 70s and that may be it.

Having a healthier senior population will do wonders for our country. With good health, many of us can continue to work and contribute positively to the economy.

At the same time, we would require less of the government. It costs much less to provide for men and women in their 70s, 80s or 90s who are healthy than it does to provide for people in their 50s or 60s who are sick.

In the long run, overall health-care costs in our country will drop, and our overburdened health-care system will become more efficient, if we as seniors spend less time in the doctors' office, the hospital or the nursing home.

Another advantage of living a healthy lifestyle is that we can set an example for those we love and care for. By living well, we can become role models for our children and grandchildren, as well as our friends and neighbors.

And there is one more reason, a spiritual one if you will, for wanting to live a healthier lifestyle.

Some years ago I was invited to speak on the subject of wellness at Rhodes College in Memphis, a school run by the Presbyterian Church. I had been a member of the college's board of directors for 20 years. The president of the school had learned of my involvement with wellness at Oklahoma State and thought it would be an appropriate subject for their weekly guest lecture series, even though most of their lectures dealt with religion.

At the end of my 45-minute talk to several hundred students and faculty and administration members, a minister in the audience raised his hand and asked what this subject had to do with religion, which is a primary focus on the campus.

I wasn't prepared for that sort of question – especially since I am of the Jewish faith. So my approach was to ask a question while I gathered my thoughts. I said, "What does it have to do with religion?" A pause. "Everything." Pause. "What is God's most precious gift?" I asked.

I didn't wait for his answer. I said, "God's most precious gift is life. He brings you into this world 99 percent of the time as a healthy child. It is not God's wish to take that healthy child's body and mind and begin a destructive process with unhealthy behavior. I think God would be pleased to know that the child pursued a healthy lifestyle and by doing so lived a long and productive life."

When you go back thousands of years, you'll note that from the beginning of time mankind was provided with everything needed to live well. The game our ancestors caught was lean from running wild. The fruits and berries they ate were untainted by pesticides. And there was no

INTRODUCTION

need for a treadmill because survival was based on being able to move quickly and stealthily in order to capture dinner.

Perhaps many years ago when we had no knowledge about what was required to stay healthy, we had an excuse. But today, there are no excuses. We know what is healthy and unhealthy.

PART I
NUTRITION

CHAPTER 1

THE IMPORTANCE OF EATING RIGHT

Learning to eat in a healthier way is the first step toward living a healthier lifestyle.

Why should you eat any differently? Well, if you're eating like most Americans, you're consuming an awful lot of foods that have been linked to health problems such as heart disease, cancer, diabetes and other ailments. Numerous studies have shown that by eating healthier, incorporated with other healthy lifestyle habits such as sufficient exercise, many people have been able to prevent these conditions from developing.

In addition, other studies have shown that simple acts, such as reducing unhealthy saturated fat in the diet, can help lower cholesterol and blood pressure, and in some instances, even reverse disease. But healthy eating isn't accomplished overnight. As we all know, the habits of a lifetime aren't so easy to change.

The important thing to realize is that this book does not provide a temporary fix to lose weight but instead outlines a process for adopting a healthy eating program – and I've tried to explain it in terms you can understand even if you don't feel you're an expert on health care

Unlike a typical diet, which so many have tried so many times only to gain the pounds back or fail to succeed at all, it isn't just about losing weight – although that usually occurs when we change to healthier ways of eating. It's also about controlling the amount and kind of food we eat so the appropriate level of weight is attained, then maintained. This is addressed later in the book in a separate section on maintaining a healthy weight.

What this section is really about is focusing – for the rest of our lives – on eating things that are good for us but still are enjoyable and eating much less of the things that aren't so good for us.

I'm here to tell you right now that healthy food doesn't have to be bland! It can be delicious, inexpensive and simple to fix in a minimum of time. With these nutrition ideas, and with the recipes in the back of the book, we show you how.

In so many instances, a healthy diet is a case of substituting more healthful food for less healthful food. I know, you're probably thinking, "But I don't want to give up steak, or stuffing and gravy, or ice cream and pecan pie, or my bagel with cream cheese, or snacks between meals."

Well, you don't have to give up enjoyable food. You simply find healthy alternatives you can enjoy as much but that improve your health instead of damaging it.

The Seretean Philosophy of Risk-Reward

Every time I eat – in fact, with everything I do – I am always consciously or subconsciously measuring risk versus reward. Is there that much pleasure in eating a high-fat, high-calorie meal or snacking on potato chips when I know of their long-term negative consequences?

Let me give you an example of how I, on rare occasions, indulge in a no-no dessert but limit the damage. Let's say I've ordered a hot-fudge sundae, which has 800 to 1,000 calories, 20 to 25 grams of saturated fat and God knows what else that's not good for me.

From that serving, which contains approximately 12 tablespoons of food, in one spoonful I've consumed 1/12, or 8 percent, of the sundae but enjoyed 30 percent of the pleasure. After five tablespoons, I've eaten 40 percent of the food and had 85 percent of the pleasure.

At that point, I say to myself, "Does it make sense to finish this and experience 60 percent of the bad stuff for only 15 percent of the pleasure?" It doesn't make sense to do that, so I put the spoon down and push away from the table.

I've received the bulk of the pleasure with less than half (only 40 percent) of the calories and saturated fat and other bad stuff. My rule is that I'm willing to taste the unhealthy but enjoyable foods of my earlier years, but I never go beyond a tasting experience.

The problem with this, of course, is that we've been taught all our lives not to waste food, to clean our plates. In fact, some of us weren't allowed to leave the table or to get dessert until the last crumb had been eaten.

To counter that, I'd like to start a "Don't Clean Your Plate Club," especially for eating out. We'll be suggesting strategies to help you in this process.

Recent studies indicate that individual portion servings in all types of restaurants have increased 50 percent in the last couple of decades.

THE IMPORTANCE OF EATING RIGHT

Years ago, on a visit to a typical fast-food restaurant, the eating experience included a hamburger, fries and a six-ounce Coke. Today, we go in for a double cheeseburger with bacon, double fries and a 16-ounce drink. So is there any surprise when you read about the U.S. having the highest overweight and obesity rates in the world?

I'd like to add that no one diet is right for everyone. What is right for me may not be perfect for you. There are so many things that have to be taken into consideration – your health when you begin, your motivation, your likes and dislikes, how sensitive your digestive system is to certain foods, spices and herbs.

I started out with the Pritikin program in 1979, which is very low in fats and was, at that time, pretty bland (that has changed over the years). Since then, I've developed my own eating program and have been revising it ever since. I've changed it as I've read hundreds of articles and books and attended additional Pritikin programs and Dr. Ornish's seminars. I revise my diet basically following the advice of these and other experts.

I make these changes, almost on a quarterly basis, to include all of the foods that new scientific evidence indicates are the healthiest. It's a continuing process and it's still evolving.

Now, let's get started by providing you with some basic knowledge to help you develop a healthier lifestyle.

CHAPTER 2
FREQUENTLY USED FOOD TERMS

Fats

Years ago, most Americans didn't worry much about fat in their diet. Meat was full of the protein needed to grow and build strong bodies. Whole milk and cookies were a great after-school snack for kids. A big helping of dessert after dinner was normal and vegetable shortenings, butter, lard, margarine and even chicken fat were used without concern.

Then research revealed that saturated fat was harmful to one's health, resulting in a proliferation of reduced fat products. Unfortunately, many of those products contained not only high levels of sugar, but also dangerous "hidden" trans fat that may have helped to raise the incidence of heart disease, diabetes, obesity and some cancers.

People do need fat; it is essential to life. It synthesizes chemicals necessary for many bodily processes, regulates cholesterol metabolism, transports and absorbs fat-soluble vitamins, contributes to healthy skin and creates energy.

Today, nutritionists and researchers know there are both "unhealthy" and "healthy" fats. Many people recognize these differences, yet still do not include enough healthy fat in their diets and/or consume too much unhealthy fat.

The major fats discussed in this book are saturated fats and trans fats – considered unhealthy – and unsaturated fats (monounsaturated fats and polyunsaturated fats) and Omega-3 oils (polyunsaturated), considered healthy.

The Unhealthy Fats

Saturated Fats

According to *The Nutrition Bible* by Jean Anderson and Barbara Deskins, an informational guide on nutrition that is used as a source book in this chapter, saturated fats are found mainly in animal products. These include meat, especially red meat such as steak and hamburgers; whole milk, ice cream, butter, cheese and some other dairy foods; and lard and chicken fat. Foods from the plant kingdom with the most saturated fat include those made with palm oil, palm kernel oil or coconut oil. The products most likely to have these oils are potato chips, french fries, non-dairy creamers, and whipped cream and toppings.

What makes saturated fat harmful? It contributes to high blood pressure, high cholesterol levels, build-up of plaque in the arteries and a variety of other problems leading to heart disease, diabetes and other serious health problems.

Trans Fats

It was only a few years ago that the federal government officially recognized the dangers from trans fat. Trans fat is created by adding hydrogen to ordinary oil to make it more solid. By the beginning of 2006, all U.S. food labels will be required to list the amount of trans fat a product contains, along with the amounts of saturated, polyunsaturated and monounsaturated fats. It is hoped this will lead most food manufacturers to eliminate trans fat from their products. Meanwhile, some food producers – those whose products don't have any trans fat – have already started including trans fat on their Nutrition Facts labels. But if it's not there, be sure to take note of the list of ingredients. If it includes partially hydrogenated oils, hydrogenated oils or vegetable shortening, that is "hidden" trans fat. The higher it is on the list, the more of it there is in the product.

Among the foods most likely to contain trans fat are fast-food items, especially french fries, fried hamburgers and donuts. Processed products are also high on the list, including many cookies and crackers, most popcorn, commercially baked cakes and pies, biscuits, some cereals, frozen fried potatoes, and frozen breaded fish and chicken. Solid margarine is also likely to contain trans fat.

Even a little trans fat is now considered by some scientists to be more unhealthy than saturated fat. Like saturated fat, it contributes to serious disease; studies have shown that it raises "bad" (LDL) cholesterol levels and lowers "good" (HDL) cholesterol levels. There are indications that it raises the triglycerides in the bloodstream and may cause platelets to stick together, increasing the chances of a blood clot.

24

The Healthy Fats

Omega-3s

Omega-3s are categorized as essential fat, that is, fat that can't be made in the body and must be obtained directly from food. Salmon, sardines, herring and other fatty fishes are all high in omega-3s, as are shellfish. Other good sources are canola and flaxseed oils, ground flaxseed, avocados, nuts – especially walnuts – non-fat and low-fat milk and cheeses, kidney beans, most soy products, eggs, melons, spinach, seaweed, wild rice and cherries, just to name a few.

Some farmed salmon has been found to have contaminants. So deep-water salmon, which is least likely to have them, is always the best choice when available. If this is of concern to you, however, you might want to limit salmon in your diet and increase intake of other sources of omega-3 oils, such as walnuts or sardines.

Omega-3 fats may truly be wonder workers. They are believed to:

• Lower the risk of heart disease by reducing the amount of cholesterol made by the liver.

• Thin blood, making clots less likely to form.

• Help regulate dangerous irregular heartbeat that can cause sudden death.

• Reduce arterial inflammation, now believed to contribute to heart attacks in people with normal cholesterol and blood pressure levels (who make up a substantial number of those who have heart attacks), as well as in those who do have high cholesterol and other heart disease risks.

• Help to reduce the risk of prostate cancer in men.

There are indications that omega-3 fats may also help prevent the complications of diabetes and arthritis, delay hunger and so help control weight, help prevent or slow down the progress of Alzheimer's disease and depression, and even reduce the incidence of autoimmune diseases, such as lupus. So, keep omega-3 fats high on your healthy food priority list.

Unsaturated Fats

Unsaturated oils – either monounsaturated or polyunsaturated – which come mainly from plant sources, also reduce the formation of arterial plaque, and oils that are primarily monounsaturated, such as olive oil, may actually increase "good" cholesterol and lower "bad" cholesterol levels.

All oils contain some saturated fat. But many vegetable oils – including canola, safflower, sunflower, olive, peanut and soybean – have high levels of unsaturated fats. They have some of both polyunsaturated and monounsaturated fats – but will usually have more of one or the other – and a relatively small amount of saturated fat. Olives, nuts and various seeds also have unsaturated fats that contribute to good health. In addition, poultry, for example, is much higher in polyunsaturated fat and lower in saturated fat than beef.

Controlling fat intake comes right behind controlling weight in the fight against serious disease. Not all "experts" agree, however, on how much fat should be ingested for good health. The USDA, for example, says it should be 30 percent or less of the total daily calorie intake for the general population, which is a big improvement over the 40 percent that is the norm in this country. I consider 30 percent a reasonable amount, although my own fat intake is closer to 20 percent of my daily menu.

Some researchers, such as Dr. Ornish, think 30 percent is far too high. In his 1993 book *Eat More and Weigh Less*, he recommended only about 10 percent fat in the daily diet, and still does in the latest version, updated in 2001. He says, however, that he has always recommended a daily dose of about 3-4 grams of fish oil, a source of omega-3 fatty acids.

On the other hand, Dr. Willett of Harvard's School of Public Health suggests in his book *Eat, Drink and Be Healthy* that about 30 percent of daily food calories as fat is perfectly OK, provided it is predominantly "healthy" fat.

FREQUENTLY USED FOOD TERMS

Cholesterol

Cholesterol has already been mentioned several times here in conjunction with fat and disease, especially heart disease. Cholesterol is a waxy, fat-like substance, but not technically a fat. *The Nutrition Bible* states that while people need it to make cell membranes, nerve sheaths and several hormones, our liver actually manufactures all most of us need. It is mainly the cholesterol and saturated fat taken in with food that contributes to health problems.

When your cholesterol tests come back to the doctor's office, overall cholesterol levels are usually broken down into triglycerides, HDL or high-density lipoproteins (the so-called "good" cholesterol) and LDL or low-density lipoproteins ("bad" cholesterol).

The job of lipoproteins – lipids (fats) plus protein – is to transport fat through the bloodstream to the appropriate destination. Lipoproteins also carry cholesterol.

Traveling with LDLs in the bloodstream, some of that cholesterol doesn't make it to where it should go. Instead, it gets into the wrong cells, especially those in the lining of blood vessels, where it can cause havoc. Once there, it's likely to be attacked by free radicals, the waste products of the blood oxidation process, which oxidize it. That can damage arteries and other cell tissues and create problems such as blood clots. So having too high a number of LDLs in your cholesterol reading can greatly increase this risk.

On the other hand, HDLs pick up and carry blood cholesterol safely to the liver, where it is eliminated or reprocessed, so generally the higher the HDL levels, the better.

Triglycerides make up most of the fat in your body, but too much of them is also considered unhealthy by most physicians and scientists. Recent studies indicate that high triglyceride levels are a contributor to heart disease.

As I mentioned earlier, when I went to the Pritikin Institute for Longevity for the first time 25 years ago, my overall cholesterol was very high, 270. Today, my overall cholesterol is much lower, my LDLs and triglyceride levels are quite low and my HDL levels are well above what is considered OK.

A healthy cholesterol level has been determined to be:

Total cholesterol	–	Under 200	–	Mine is 135
HDL	–	Above 40	–	Mine is 61
LDL	–	Under 130	–	Mine is 64
Triglyceride	–	Under 150	–	Mine is 52

While too much unhealthy fat is the main culprit in raising blood cholesterol levels, physicians generally advise patients to limit their intake of foods that have a lot of cholesterol, such as eggs. But with the exception of their cholesterol level, eggs are now considered pretty healthy, although an overall weekly average of no more than one a day usually is recommended for people with normal cholesterol levels, and fewer or none for those with elevated levels. I prefer to use only egg whites or egg substitutes. Some shellfish, especially shrimp, also contain a lot of cholesterol but their omega-3 benefits outweigh the negative effects.

Proteins

Every part of the human body is built from protein. People need it on a regular basis because humans can't store excess protein like they do fat, nor can they store amino acids, the building blocks of protein. Amino acids are needed for growth, repair and maintenance of the body and to make enzymes, hormones and antibodies.

Egg white, meat, poultry, fish, non-fat milk, non-fat cheese and other non-fat dairy products are some of the best animal sources of protein. Soy, dried beans, peanut butter, rice, whole grains, corn, lima beans and other plant products are also just a few of the many protein sources.

While there has been no decision among the experts on whether one kind of protein is better than the other, there have been some indications that plant proteins are related to lower rates of heart disease, while animal proteins are related to higher rates of heart disease. While protein itself doesn't appear to have a relationship with cancer rates, frying and grilling meat very well done is believed to activate certain carcinogens. However, there are few research findings to determine whether or not this is actually harmful to human beings.

One of the most important things about protein is what else is included in the package. Healthy protein has low saturated fat and no trans fat, a fair amount of unsaturated fat, including, as in the case of some seafood, healthy omega-3 fats. Healthy plant proteins are good sources of fiber and unsaturated fats, including omega-3s in some instances, and are replete with antioxidants, vitamins and minerals.

Carbohydrates

Carbohydrates are sugars and starches that provide fuel for the body. There are three kinds of carbohydrates:

- **Simple sugars** – fructose (sugar from fruit); glucose (blood sugar), sugar found in the bloodstream; or galactose, usually found in combination with other simple sugars.

- **Double sugars** – a pair of simple sugars, such as the combination of glucose and fructose, which forms sucrose (table sugar).

- **Complex carbohydrates** – complicated chains of glucose molecules.

All of these carbohydrates are broken down in the body into glucose (blood sugar), which provides energy to cells. It is believed that most simple and double sugars usually break down into a usable form very quickly, while most complex carbohydrates usually take a longer time to break down, especially if the food source also contains fiber.

Studies have indicated, however, that not all simple sugars are digested quickly and not all complex carbohydrates are digested slowly. For example, a white potato, considered a complex carbohydrate, is believed to be digested very rapidly.

How can the rapid digestion of sugars and starches cause problems in the body? When the body is rapidly flooded with glucose, it may be excessive. This can trigger a rush of energy but also trigger the pancreas to produce enough insulin to rapidly lower blood sugar. That rush of energy can be followed by a period of low energy. Although studies have not yet shown a direct connection between blood sugar levels dropping and hunger, it is believed by many scientists that this process can produce hunger cravings in order to try to get you back to a higher energy level.

The job of the pancreas is to release insulin, which controls blood sugar. It removes any excess and stores it in appropriate parts of the body, releasing it when blood sugar gets too low. But when it runs out of appropriate space to store the excess, it is stored in the fat cells, and becomes a major contributor to weight gain.

In addition, a high-sugar diet and constant repetition of the high to low to high blood sugar cycle may cause the overworked pancreas to get out of whack – which could mean it doesn't control insulin levels, consequently the amount of blood sugar, very well. That could lead eventually to chronic hypoglycemia (low blood sugar) or possibly even to insulin resistance, which can occur when the body stops responding to insulin the way it should. These in turn may lead to Type 2 diabetes (previously called "adult onset" diabetes), when instead of being stored in cells, blood sugar can be excreted in the urine, depriving the body of fuel. Eventually, the pancreas may stop producing any insulin at all.

This repetitive process does not cause Type 1 diabetes, an autoimmune disease once called "juvenile diabetes" because of its typical onset in childhood. It can, however, cause higher triglyceride, lower HDLs, and other problems leading to heart disease.

Some of the culprits in this process are whole milk (which contains lactose, that is, milk sugar), white and brown sugars, molasses and syrups, sodas (soft drinks), honey, candy and many other sweets and desserts, pizza and pancakes.

Most complex carbohydrates, however, appear to take longer to turn into glucose in most people – unless they are diabetics, who process glucose differently than people who aren't diabetic. Consequently, smaller amounts of sugar are likely to be released over a longer period, creating a more stable form of energy. This process may reduce many of the risks contributing to a variety of serious illnesses. Good sources of complex carbohydrates are apples, peas, beans and whole grains.

Unfortunately, most of the grains we eat in this country have been processed or refined; that is, the high-carbohydrate part is separated from the parts that have most of the vitamins, minerals and unsaturated fat. In other words, most of the "good stuff" is gone.

The government requires refined foods to be enriched – that is, some of the lost vitamins and minerals are put back in. But enriched foods still lack some of the missing vitamins and minerals and usually still lack fiber as well. So it's best to choose grains such as brown rice, 100 percent whole wheat (stone ground is best) or other whole-grain breads, flour, cereals and pasta. Stay away from refined grains like white flour, white bread, white pasta and white rice. Some whole-grain cereals are especially good choices because they have been fortified; that is, while they haven't lost any valuable nutrients through processing, even more vitamins, minerals and/or fiber have been added.

Fiber

Although dietary fiber is classified as a complex carbohydrate, it doesn't have any calories, vitamins or minerals. But it is still very important to good health.

Scientists have been trying to define fiber since 1929, when it was called "unavailable carbohydrate." Basically though, fiber is plant material we eat that we can't digest but that is still important for good health.

Today's scientific thinking classifies fiber as both "dietary" and "added."

Dietary fiber is that which occurs naturally in the food we eat. Added fiber is added in some way to food, either by being extracted from plants, created synthetically or modified.

There are two kinds of fiber: water-soluble and water-insoluble. Water-soluble fiber adds bulk to our diet and helps to lower cholesterol and stabilize the amount of glucose circulating in the bloodstream by slowing down the digestion of other carbohydrates. Oatmeal, oat bran, dried peas and beans, apples and citrus fruits are among the best sources. Water-insoluble fiber doesn't do anything until it gets to our colon and intestines, where it promotes good health as it passes through them.

It may not be a good idea to switch to a high-fiber diet too rapidly if you're used to just a little fiber in your diet, because that may cause problems such as gas, diarrhea and bloating. Blended products, such as pasta made from part whole-grain flour and part refined flour, can ease people into a higher-fiber diet. It's also important to drink plenty of water with additional fiber to avoid irritation or more serious problems in the digestive tract. However, people with diverticulosis should avoid eating too much fiber.

Eating a wide variety of fruits, vegetables and whole grains will provide both kinds of fiber in the diet, which is what most nutritionists recommend.

FREQUENTLY USED FOOD TERMS

Antioxidants and Phytochemicals

Antioxidants are chemicals in foods that are believed to protect proteins, DNA and other important compounds in the body, along with tissues and cells, by neutralizing free radicals. The damage caused by free radicals speeds up the aging process and contributes to the development of cataracts, cancers, heart disease, memory loss and many other health problems.

The most familiar antioxidants include the vitamins C and E, the minerals selenium and manganese, and carotenoids, the plant pigments that give fruits and vegetables color, such as lycopene, which makes tomatoes red.

Each antioxidant has its own chemical properties and works a little differently than the others. There are many things that are unknown about antioxidants, but numerous studies are under way to try to find out more about how they work in the body. Indications so far are that they seem to work best in conjunction with one another – that is, they work well in foods in which a number of them are combined, especially the B vitamins. The best sources of antioxidants are fruits and vegetables, especially deep-colored ones such as blueberries and watermelon, and spinach, kale, carrots, oranges, sweet potatoes, tomatoes and broccoli.

There are hundreds of thousands of phytochemicals, compounds from plants, which are neither truly vitamin nor mineral, found mainly in fruits and vegetables. Some antioxidants are also phytochemicals. Believed to aid in fighting cancer, some also may help in lowering cholesterol and reducing or preventing other health problems. Only a comparatively few phytochemicals have been thoroughly studied, but many more studies are under way. An example of a phytochemical is catechins – found in green tea, strawberries and other berries – which is believed to crank up the immune system and reduce the risk of gastrointestinal cancers.

Calories

Food calories are actually a measurement of energy. Fat has more calories (9 per gram) than protein or carbohydrates (4 calories each per gram). But for the most part, calories, no matter what the source, are all digested at about the same pace.

Calories do make a difference. After all, at the end of the day, if you take in more calories than you use up, you will gain weight.

FREQUENTLY USED FOOD TERMS

How many calories are too much? The answer is an individual one that depends on a number of factors. Among these are your body frame (small, medium or large), current weight and height, gender, age and activity level, not to mention the diversified opinions of a variety of experts and the proliferation of charts created by different agencies, organizations, physicians and nutritionists. There are other important factors that make a difference too, such as portion size and how the calories you eat are prepared or processed.

If you have gained weight and want to lose it, one approach is to keep a record of the calories you've consumed over a period of time. To supplement the calorie information found on food labels, I suggest you pick up a book that contains information on the number of calories in servings of foods that don't have labels, such as fresh fruit and poultry. These are available at just about any grocery store at a modest price, usually at the checkout counter.

Be sure to figure out the actual number of portions you're eating at a time by checking the Nutrition Facts panel on food labels. According to the portion sizes shown on the nutrition panel, you'll often find you're eating more than one, perhaps even two or three. Then add up the calories ingested each day. Chances are you'll be surprised by your total calorie intake!

Do you still really need to count calories these days? I don't really recommend that on a regular basis because when you start eating healthier, low-fat and low-sugar foods in more moderate portions, chances are good that you will greatly reduce the number of calories you take in daily. It's certainly an option if you find it the easiest way to keep tabs on your diet, but it can be a time-consuming job. Basically, it's eating healthy and exercising that are vital to controlling your weight.

CHAPTER 3

VITAMINS AND MINERALS

Vitamins and minerals are integral to the health of human beings, and most can be found in ample amounts in a well-balanced diet. Following are lists of the most important vitamins and minerals, what they do, and the best food sources for each one. This chapter also includes information about multivitamins and multimineral supplements, as well as specific vitamin and mineral supplements.

Vitamins

Vitamins are organic substances, or those that come from living organisms. They're nutrients the body needs.

Vitamin A

The work of vitamin A is to build immunity and fight infection; help to synthesize protein; aid in bone growth, healthy skin and sexual function; fight the damage caused by air pollution; help the gall bladder function; and especially to aid eyesight, in particular to ward off night blindness.

Some vitamin A comes from animal-based foods such as milk, cheese and eggs. However, they should be eaten in moderation because of their high saturated fat content, unless, as in the case of dairy products, they are either non-fat or low-fat. Reducing fat content does not reduce the vitamins in foods.

According to *The American Vegetarian Cookbook* by Marilyn Diamond, which lists information about vitamins and minerals in addition to recipes, the best vegetable sources are carrots, collards and kale, dandelion and hot (red) peppers. There are numerous other good vegetable sources too; among them: leafy green vegetables such as spinach and lettuce, beet greens, asparagus, broccoli, chives, sweet red peppers, pumpkin and winter squash such as acorn, butternut or Hubbard.

Good fruit sources are mangos, cantaloupe, peaches, prunes, sour cherries, nectarines, fresh and dried apricots, and papaya.

Vitamin B1, Thiamine (thiamin)

This vitamin helps provide a healthy nervous system; promotes growth, muscle building (including the heart), cell oxidation and liver health; increases the appetite; and helps in the digestion of carbohydrates.

The best sources are all whole grains, but especially millet, whole wheat and brown rice; legumes; nuts, mainly pecans and pine nuts; and sunflower and sesame seeds. Good vegetables for vitamin B1 include asparagus, bamboo shoots, broccoli, Brussels sprouts, leafy green vegetables, sweet potatoes and garlic. Good fruit sources include oranges, pineapple, prunes and raisins. There are no animal sources.

Vitamin B2, Riboflavin

Riboflavin helps metabolize fats and protein, keep kidneys and the heart in good shape, and promote creation of red blood cells and antibodies. It's necessary for healthy hair, eyes, skin, nails and liver, and it improves resistance to disease.

The best sources include almonds, cashews, chestnuts, wild rice and wheat germ. Other very good sources are hot (red) peppers, along with other vegetables like mushrooms, pumpkin, parsley, spinach and turnip greens. Good fruit sources include prunes, dried peaches and dried bananas. Whole grains, rice, wheat bran, legumes, and sesame and sunflower seeds are also very good at supplying riboflavin.

From the animal world, the best sources are oily fish such as flounder and salmon, as well as mussels, crabs and pork. Other sources are non-fat yogurt and skim milk.

Vitamin B3, Niacin

Niacin is necessary for converting carbohydrates, fats and protein into energy. It also helps people maintain health in the digestive tract, skin and nerves. Unlike most other water-soluble vitamins, it isn't destroyed by heat or light, but like them, it can leach out in cooking water.

Our bodies can make niacin from the amino acid tryptophan. The best food sources are turkey and other poultry, whole grains, legumes, lean meat, oily fish, avocados, dates, figs, prunes and peanut butter.

Vitamin B5, Pantothenic Acid

This vitamin, perhaps less familiar to people than some of the other Bs, has important work to do. It promotes production of antibodies; contributes to healthy skin, hair and adrenal function; helps in handling stress; aids in liver health; and helps to develop the central nervous system and build cells.

The best sources are sunflower seeds, buckwheat flour, wheat germ, papaya and legumes. Green vegetables such as cabbage, broccoli, artichokes, celery and kale and whole grains like buckwheat and whole wheat provide other good sources. So do chicken, brewer's yeast, eggs and nuts.

Vitamin B6, Pyridoxine

This vitamin helps the body digest and assimilate food, promotes production of insulin and adrenaline, helps produce antibodies and red blood cells, prevents nausea, and may assist in controlling weight.

The best sources are whole grains, especially buckwheat and wheat germ; cabbage and most other green leafy vegetables; beets, green peppers, and carrots. Good fruit sources are oranges, lemons, bananas, papayas, avocados and cantaloupes. Other substantial sources of vitamin B6 include walnuts, filberts, sunflower seeds, and legumes, especially red beans, pinto beans, white beans and split peas. Beef, turkey and fish are also good sources.

Vitamin B9, Folic Acid

Folic acid is necessary for cell growth, helps the body form red blood cells and produce antibodies, and is important for processing protein.

The best vegetable sources are asparagus, beet greens, broccoli, dark green leafy vegetables such as endive and spinach, Swiss chard, kale, lima beans, mushrooms and turnips. Nuts, nutritional yeast and wheat germ are also good sources of folic acid.

Vitamin B12, Cobalamin

Vitamin B12 is responsible for the formation and maintenance of the nervous system and the formation of red blood cells. Children need it for growth, and it blocks degeneration of the nerve cells and helps the body metabolize carbohydrates.

Although some plant products eaten by vegans (people who eat no animal products), especially certain seaweed and algae, do contain vitamin B12, no research has indicated that humans can really access this form of it. There are also questions as to whether it is the same B12 found in animal products. So far, the research hasn't turned up any safe plant sources to obtain vitamin B12, so at least for now, the best sources of it are animal products like lean meat, non-fat yogurt, and eggs.

Vitamin B12 sometimes becomes hard to digest and use, especially as people age. A lack of sufficient B12 can cause pernicious anemia, as well as fatigue and lack of balance. To remedy this problem of not being able to absorb B12, patients may be given periodic injections of the vitamin. In addition, some physicians prescribe high doses of B12, often along with folic acid and vitamin B6, in a pill form.

The B-complex

The B-complex usually refers to the B vitamins when they are found together in the same foods and have some related functions to each other. Together, they are important for the normal function of the nervous system, to provide energy and help keep the digestive system working properly. Included in this category are: thiamine, riboflavin, niacin, folic acid, pantothenic acid, vitamin B6 and vitamin B12, and biotin (vitamin H), which is also considered part of the B-complex.

Deficiencies in three B-complex vitamins, folic acid and vitamins B6 and B12, have been linked to high levels of homocysteine, a protein byproduct. Homocysteine is believed to contribute to inflammation of the blood vessels, a factor that can lead to heart disease. These three B vitamins help change homocysteine into amino acids that are not damaging. Two of the main foods that supply all the B-complex vitamins together are whole-grain cereals and brewer's yeast.

Vitamin C, Ascorbic Acid

This vitamin prevents infection and promotes healing; fights the negative effects of smoke and pollution; helps prevent hemorrhaging; promotes healthy gums and bones and healthy formation of connective tissue and teeth; helps regulate cholesterol; helps maintain healthy sex organs and adrenal glands; and shores up capillary tissue. Physical stress can create the need for additional vitamin C.

37

VITAMINS AND MINERALS

The sources of vitamin C are all plant based. The best are citrus fruits like fresh oranges and lemons and their juices, and tangerines; also strawberries, guava and black currents. Tomatoes, broccoli, Brussels sprouts, sweet red and green bell peppers, spinach and kale, kohlrabi, watercress, and hot red and green peppers are also very good sources of vitamin C.

Vitamin D

Ultraviolet rays change ergosterol (an oily substance on our skin) into vitamin D, very important in regulating the use of phosphorous in the body, and especially important in regulating the use of calcium. Vitamin D is also necessary for a healthy nervous system and strong teeth and bones, and it protects against muscle weakness, assists thyroid function and blood clotting and, through calcium absorption, helps to regulate the heart.

The best source is sunshine. But wearing sunscreen may block it out and it can be difficult to get enough sunshine in winter in Northern climates. Fortunately, there are some good food sources, such as papaya and raspberries. Vitamin D is sometimes added to calcium supplements for people who need additional calcium. Other good sources are fish liver oils and fish like tuna, sardines, trout and salmon; and non-fat milk and other non-fat or reduced-fat dairy products with added vitamin D.

Vitamin E

This is a potent antioxidant that also helps to keep blood cells healthy and improve circulation; helps the body prevent blood clots, protect lungs against air pollution and absorb selenium and phosphorous; helps keep the reproductive system healthy; is necessary in order for muscles to use oxygen; and prevents sterility.

Good sources are sesame and sunflower seeds; nuts; barley, brown rice and other whole grains, and wheat germ; and asparagus, watercress, spinach and broccoli, leeks and sweet potatoes. Good fruit sources are blackberries and pears. Other sources include lean meats, milk, eggs and molasses.

Vitamin H, Biotin

Biotin helps to metabolize carbohydrates, proteins and unsaturated fatty acids, utilize the B vitamins, and maintain bone marrow, skin, hair and sex glands. It's important for normal growth and for the health of the kidneys, liver and pancreas.

Good sources are brown rice, soy flour, oats and wheat bran; spinach, kale, endive and asparagus; cauliflower, mushrooms; and brewer's yeast.

Minerals

Minerals are inorganic elements – that is, they aren't formed from plants or animals – and there are several hundred of them. The body only needs a handful of these to maintain good health, however.

The main seven minerals the body needs, sometimes called macrominerals, are calcium, chlorine (chloride), phosphorus, magnesium, potassium, sodium and sulfur.

Microminerals, also known as trace minerals or trace elements, are just as important as macrominerals but are only necessary in tiny quantities for good health. Some of these are chromium, copper, iodine, iron, manganese, nickel, selenium, zinc and boron.

The most important minerals are listed below along with their functions and listings of the best sources for each one.

Calcium

We all know calcium builds strong teeth and bones, but it also helps to regulate heart rhythm and normalize metabolism, strengthens our nervous system, helps blood to clot and muscles to work, and activates certain enzymes.

There are numerous sources of calcium in addition to milk and other dairy products. The best among them are dried figs, apples, peaches and both dried and fresh bananas; and almonds, Brazil nuts and filberts. Good vegetable sources are seaweed, broccoli, turnip greens, all kinds of squash, artichokes, Brussels sprouts, cabbages of various kinds, spinach and kale. Other good sources include whole grains, legumes – especially tofu and miso from soybeans – and sesame seeds; and fish eaten with the bones, such as canned salmon and sardines.

VITAMINS AND MINERALS

Iron

Iron helps to form hemoglobin, which carries oxygen from the lungs to body cells. It promotes resistance to disease and increases energy, and it contributes to healthy bone, brain and muscle.

Excellent sources are whole grains, especially wheat and rice bran, and wheat germ; fruits, especially dried figs and apricots, dates, prunes and raisins; vegetables such as spinach and squash; tofu and most legumes and nuts; and blackstrap molasses. Oily fish and mussels also supply iron.

Magnesium

This important mineral assists in the metabolism of vitamin C and calcium; helps keep the body in alkaline-acid balance; stimulates elimination; helps the body utilize fats; and promotes healthy arteries, heart, bones, nerves, muscles and teeth.

The best sources are whole grains, such as millet and whole wheat, and especially wheat bran and wheat germ; legumes, especially lima beans; fruits, especially figs and bananas, and apples, dates, avocados and apricots; vegetables, including garlic, spinach and corn; almonds and cashews; and shellfish, particularly shrimp.

Phosphorous

Phosphorous works with calcium to promote growth of bones and teeth, and to metabolize fats and carbohydrates. It helps grow and repair cells and nerves; aids healthy activity of muscles; and is needed to provide energy. It is also very important in maintaining the correct acid-alkaline balance within the body.

There are dozens of great sources of phosphorous. Among them: all kinds of whole grains, especially rice and wheat bran, and wheat germ, and others such as barley and millet; almonds, walnuts, Brazil and pine nuts; sesame and pumpkin seeds; legumes, especially soybeans, pinto beans, red beans and white beans. Other sources are all kinds of fruits, especially dried apricots, apples and peaches; and vegetables such as garlic, yams, artichokes and mushrooms. Almost all meat, poultry and fish supply phosphorus; in fact, anything with protein has it.

40

Potassium

Potassium assists in regulating heartbeat and helps prevent nervous and muscular irritability, such as leg cramps. It helps kidneys detoxify the blood; helps maintain the pH balance in blood and tissues; stimulates endocrine hormone production; aids in elimination; and helps the body avoid and reduce raised blood pressure by ridding it of too much sodium.

The best sources are bananas, apricots, and dried apples; other fruits, including dates, nectarines, grapefruit and oranges; dried soy; almonds; Mung and lima beans; and rice and wheat bran. Vegetables are also good choices, including broccoli, Brussels sprouts, carrots, celery, fennel, radishes, spinach and various squash.

Selenium

Selenium has an antioxidant effect similar to that of vitamin E and helps to clean up free radicals. It also preserves the elasticity of tissues and helps the healthy function of testicles.

The best sources are whole grains, especially wheat germ, and rice and wheat bran; and vegetables such as broccoli, mushrooms, garlic, onions, kelp, asparagus and cabbage. Other good sources are a variety of fruits, such as apples, cantaloupe, grapefruit, honeydew melon, raspberries and pineapple. Legumes and nuts, especially Brazil nuts, also supply selenium.

Sodium

Although people are encouraged to limit sodium (salt) intake, especially if they have high blood pressure, the fact is that sodium is necessary for our bodies to maintain life. Working with potassium, it regulates the flow of fluids in and out of individual cells. Also classified as an electrolyte, it is necessary for metabolizing protein and carbohydrates, sparking nerve impulses and maintaining the body's acid/alkali balance.

It's pretty hard to be sodium deficient in this country. People do obtain some through a few foods naturally high in sodium but get it mainly from the substantial amounts of salt added to canned and processed food and from salt used in cooking or at the table. The only people likely to be deficient are those who run marathons or who use diuretics on a regular basis. Generally, the deficiency is only temporary and can be remedied quickly.

Zinc

Zinc assists in healing wounds and burns, helps metabolize protein and carbohydrates, assists in the function of the prostate gland and contributes to healthy reproductive organs, helps transfer carbon dioxide from tissues to lungs, is necessary in order to form DNA, and is also very important for the health of the brain, kidneys, liver and thyroid.

The best sources include sesame, pumpkin and sunflower seeds; most nuts; tofu, mushrooms, green peas, spinach and to a lesser degree other leafy green vegetables, lentils, lima beans, cornmeal and the outer coating of whole grains. The best animal sources include oysters and other shellfish as well as lean meat.

Specific Vitamin and Mineral Supplements

Physicians may recommend certain vitamin and/or mineral supplements for specific problems, such as calcium tablets for those at risk for osteoporosis. Often these work in conjunction with other vitamins or minerals. For example, vitamin D helps the body absorb calcium, so the two are often combined in one pill.

Rely on your doctor to recommend which vitamins and minerals, if needed, should be taken and in what amounts. For example, large doses of niacin shouldn't be taken as a supplement without medical direction because it can be dangerous. In addition, too much vitamin A in supplemental form can draw calcium from the bones. This does not happen with natural vitamin A from food sources.

Be sure to tell your doctor what medications and supplements you're already taking to avoid the chance of drug interactions.

Certain individuals might receive particular benefits from specific vitamin and/or mineral supplements. They may also benefit from unrefined foods (not enriched, refined products) that have been fortified with additional vitamins and minerals, such as fortified whole-grain cereals. These groups include:

- People who don't spend much time outdoors, so don't get enough vitamin D from sunshine.
- Seniors, who often have trouble absorbing vitamin B12.
- Vegans – people who eat no animal products and may not get enough vitamin B12, some other vitamins, and complete protein.

- People with certain gastrointestinal disorders.
- Those with serious medical problems such as cancer.

Multivitamins/Minerals

There are both multivitamin supplements and multivitamin/multimineral supplements, which are what most people take. These nutritional supplements include varying percentages of most of the vitamins and minerals necessary to sustain good health.

Ideally, all the vitamins and minerals we need would come from food. A lot of people, however, do not take in enough of these important nutrients on a regular basis. Studies have shown that taking multivitamins regularly can reduce the risk of serious disease. Consequently, many physicians recommend that their patients take daily multiple vitamins and mineral supplements as an insurance policy. On my doctor's advice, I take Centrum Silver, a multivitamin/multi-mineral supplement designed for people over 50.

A word to the wise about herbal and plant supplements: be sure to consult your doctor, or at least a good nutritionist, rather than taking them on your own. Unlike food, the Food and Drug Administration (FDA) does not closely regulate these supplements, which include vitamins and minerals. Although supplement manufacturers must be able to back up specific health claims, be especially careful of those that imply they will energize you, make you smarter or improve memory, and especially those that suggest they can help you lose weight. A number of these claims have been disproved or have not been verified. And some supplements may not be safe, particularly in large amounts.

CHAPTER 4

SALT

Why Salt Matters

Salt is critical to human life because it helps the body retain fluids. Although we need only a very small amount of salt, it is essential for us in order to have enough plasma, the fluid part of blood. Without it, bodily fluids would lose water, blood pressure would drop dramatically, complete dehydration would set in and we would die.

All animals, including human beings, are physiologically attuned to recognize this and automatically seek salt when it's needed.

Lower Salt Levels Recommended

You won't see it on the food label yet, but the latest dietary guidelines have dramatically changed the government's standard for how much salt Americans should have in their daily diets. According to a report from Harvard's School of Public Health, the new guidelines from the Institute of Medicine, which sets the standards for nutrients in the U.S., recommend that people lower their sodium (salt) intake to 1,500 milligrams (mg.) per day. That's down from the government's previous recommendation of 2,400 mg. daily by about 40 percent. The guidelines were published by the Department of Health and Human Services and the Department of Agriculture on January 12, 2005.

Making the change won't be easy. The guidelines not only change the government's previous recommended level of sodium, according to the Harvard report, they also suggest an even more drastic reduction in the amount the average American actually consumes every day – which is anywhere from 3,500 to 4,000 mg. daily.

Why the concern? Essentially, excess salt can raise the volume of blood, which can then stimulate certain hormones to raise blood pressure. Although other factors such as weight and exercise play a role, the more salt consumed, generally the higher the blood pressure. Lower salt intake and, generally, blood pressure drops.

Most researchers agree that chronic high blood pressure,

hypertension, increases the risks not only of heart disease and stroke, but also kidney disease.

Lowering Salt Can Lower Blood Pressure

The first known researcher to link salt intake to high blood pressure was Dr. Lewis Dahl in 1972. From his research, he concluded high salt intake does contribute to hypertension, chronic and persistent high blood pressure.

A study in the late 1990s called Dietary Approaches to Stop Hypertension (DASH-Sodium), however, definitely showed that reducing salt in the diet could also help reduce blood pressure levels. Supported by the National Heart, Lung and Blood Institute, the study took place in several research facilities around the country and was presented by Harvard researchers in May 2000.

The study compared people on the DASH diet – a lower-fat, high-fiber, high-potassium diet moderately low in dairy foods – with others on a "typical" American diet in three categories: high, medium and low salt intake. All the subjects in the study improved their blood pressure levels on the healthy diet, even those with the highest salt intake, including those with hypertension. The lower the salt intake, though, the lower the blood pressure. Those who fared the best were the hypertensive people who restricted their dietary salt the most, substantially decreasing their chances of a heart attack or a stroke.

The study also showed that lowering your salt intake appears to be especially helpful in reducing blood pressure in people who are overweight and/or are older. As seniors, this is important to know.

Why Do We Do It and What Can We Do About It?

About one-fourth of our taste buds are dedicated to recognizing salt.

So, since the body knows when it's necessary, why do we Americans consume so much salt when we don't really need much of it and too much can be bad for us? Basically, it's because food manufacturers use it for a variety of purposes, such as creating a certain texture in their products, so we're used to its taste. Food companies recognize this, so they continue to put salt into our food in high volume. We buy these products and get even more used to it, and the cycle continues.

The idea of eliminating salt is repugnant to many people. Food without salt or made with little salt just seems too blah and downright unappealing, both boring and a destroyer of the flavor of the foods they enjoy.

However, our lust for salt is an acquired taste – it's not natural. Therefore, it is possible to acquire different tastes, eventually eliminating our "addiction" to high-salt products. At some point, people who've had to lower or even eliminate salt in their diets often lose their taste for it because they are now actually experiencing the real taste of many foods for the first time. I have almost no salt in my diet and I don't miss it at all.

One way to get this re-education of the taste buds is to learn to substitute other ingredients for salt. Lemon, lime, vinegar, low-salt mustard and ketchup, and Italian seasoning – which includes herbs such as garlic, oregano, and parsley – will all add flavor to everyday meals. Low-sodium soy sauce is a good substitute. Use fresh herbs and spices every time you can because they have more flavor than dried herbs. Ginger is one of the best. Ordinary Dijon mustard is low in salt but adds zest, and cayenne pepper helps to bring out the naturally salty taste in many foods. The recipes at the end of the book incorporate most of these seasoning ideas.

Try to drink fresh juices and eat fruits and vegetables whenever possible. They're not only naturally low in salt, but they're also good for you, as you already know.

Reducing salt intake can be difficult. So start now by putting away the saltshaker. If I have guests at my home for dinner, they have to request it. The shaker is never on the table.

Then eliminate salt altogether in cooking. This is a good start, but the real villain is not the salt you add, it's the often hidden salt in processed, canned, frozen and restaurant food that is responsible for 80 percent of our salt intake. If you totaled up all of the salt consumed in these foods for just one day, you'd be shocked at how much goes into your system on a regular basis.

For example, according to information cited in *Eat Healthy and Live*, Dr. Willett shows that the average amount of sodium in a cup of canned chili with beans is about 1,336 mg. Think what that means. At that rate, under the new sodium guidelines of 1,500 mg. daily, you would have consumed almost all of your daily allowance with one dish of food.

Here are some average sodium levels of a few other high-salt culprits shown on Dr. Willett's list, which came from *The New England Journal of Medicine Heart Watch* of December 1997. While some of these numbers have probably changed since then, chances are they haven't gotten any lower.

- A cup of macaroni and cheese, a whopping 1,343 mg.
- Three ounces of corned beef brisket, 964 mg.
- One 4-gram chicken bouillon cube – a staple for many cooks – 743 mg.
- A cup of raisin bran, 428 mg. – who would suspect?
- One cup of canned green beans, another surprise at 354 mg.
- A cup of canned peas, 408 mg.
- One-half cup of regular pasta sauce, 515 mg.
- A medium-sized blueberry muffin, 255 mg.

So a dinner of brisket and a serving of canned green beans, without anything else, equals 1,318 mg. Not much left over for dessert or much of anything later in the day.

It will probably take several years for the latest government dietary recommendations on sodium to be added to food labels, and even longer for food producers to respond and bring down the amount of salt in their products. So read the labels now, think about the revised dietary guidelines, and avoid foods with high salt levels, because it's better to be safe than sorry.

Dos and Don'ts to Reduce Salt Intake

- Do start to reduce salt in your diet.

- Don't indulge in fast-food products, junk food and processed foods, which generally are very high in salt.

- Don't eat salted nuts and seeds.

- Don't put your saltshaker on the table. Reserve it for guests who request it.

SALT

- Do eat plenty of fresh vegetables and drink fresh juices – most are naturally low in salt.

- Do use spices, herbs and other seasonings as substitutes for salt to bring out full flavor.

- Do read the labels on canned goods, frozen goods and prepackaged baked goods for salt content.

- Do learn to enjoy the natural taste of food.

CHAPTER 5

WATER, WATER, WATER –
AND OTHER BEVERAGES

Water

For years, we've been told to drink eight 8-ounce glasses of water a day, an amount that many people find difficult to swallow. But one thing seems certain: most people do not drink nearly enough. Water is absolutely essential for life. Humans may live for a long time with little or no food, but usually cannot live more than a few days at most without water.

Some studies indicate many people are so unaccustomed to drinking water that they no longer recognize thirst. They may actually think they are hungry instead. But as a matter of fact, water can assuage hunger, as it can help fill you up.

My target is to drink eight 8-ounce glasses of water every day, but I know some days I may drink less. So I understand the difficulty of trying to drink that much, but it's a constant goal. If you can't drink eight, drink as much as you can. The more you can drink, the better off you will be. I drink as much as I can, especially during and after exercise.

What is it that makes water so important? Well, first it replenishes the water in our body lost by sweating and urination. It helps us digest our food and flushes out impurities. It can also flush out excess fat. It nourishes and bathes our tissues and organs and helps body cells do their job. And it fills you up with zero calories.

One way to drink enough water is to carry a water bottle with you. You've probably already noticed the number of people who do this has greatly increased over the past decade or so. Just fill a bottle, water jug or even a thermos with ordinary tap water or buy bottled water. If you don't like the taste of the water from your tap, you can put a water filter system on your spigot to filter out unpleasant taste, minerals and possible impurities.

The benefit of keeping a water bottle handy is two-fold: first, you have readily accessible water to drink all day long because, even if you run out, more water will be available almost any place you go. If you're traveling, it can keep you from having to make a stop, even at a drive-through, to buy a carbonated drink when you get thirsty. This is important not only in terms of time and money, but because many people tend to use carbonated sodas in place of water. These beverages are often high in calories, caffeine and sugars and do nothing to nourish your body.

Among the latest findings are indications that water may actually help people to lose weight. Preliminary findings by German researchers have found that drinking water speeds up the rate at which people burn up calories. The subjects were healthy men and women who were tested after drinking only 17 ounces. It only took about 10 minutes for their metabolisms to begin to speed up. During a 30- to 40-minute period, their metabolisms increased by an average of 30 percent.

Coffee and Tea

Most people seldom think about it, but they often are ingesting a lot more caffeine than they realize. Caffeine is everywhere, not only in beverages like coffee and tea, but in carbonated colas, chocolate milk, candy bars, cookies and cocoa. Unlike many other food ingredients, you'll never find out how much caffeine is in a beverage, or even in foods, for that matter, because it isn't required to be listed on the label.

But what's the harm, you ask, of drinking a cup or two of coffee to help you wake up in the morning? Probably not much, as long as it is limited to a few cups and you're not taking in a lot of additional caffeine from other sources throughout the day.

Believe it or not, caffeine is one of the most widely used mood-enhancing drugs in the world. The problem with coffee is that it is loaded with caffeine, and like many other drugs, caffeine for some people is addictive. The more you drink, the more you want.

This is because caffeine in large amounts can cause the release of the hormones that cause the liver to release stored blood sugar rapidly, leading to elevated blood sugar. This usually creates a temporary rush but it may be more sugar than the body can handle at one time. This, in turn, can increase the release of insulin, which may then lower blood sugar too much, leading to an energy drain and perhaps the craving for more coffee.

These reactions, occurring too frequently over a long period of time, can contribute to health problems. This is a reason diabetics are often advised to drink only decaffeinated beverages or at least limit their intake of regular coffee.

In addition, caffeine raises blood pressure and the release of hormones that prepare the body for stressful situations. It's true that coffee contributes to mental alertness, at least for a time. But drinking too many cups of coffee isn't recommended because caffeine has other negative side effects. It can irritate the digestive system, especially the stomach, and cause diarrhea. It can deplete the body of certain vitamins and minerals, among them most of the B vitamins, especially B12. It can also leech calcium from the bones, increasing the risk of osteoporosis. Caffeine can cause rapid heartbeat, nervousness and dizziness, and it can increase stress.

While coffee contains more caffeine by far than any other beverage Americans drink, it is not the only culprit. People who drink numerous glasses of strong iced tea or cups of hot tea daily may have similar reactions: addiction to the caffeine, rapid increases and losses of energy, and insulin and hormones racing through their bloodstream that may lead to health problems. Decaffeinated coffee and tea, however, will negate most of the side effects of caffeine.

Other Beverages

If you think about it, you probably know other folks, especially younger people, who always seem to have a soda in their hands. Chances are good that, in most instances, these are not caffeine-free drinks, even if they are sugar-free.

Too much caffeine from any source can have negative side effects, so I don't drink coffee or any other beverage with caffeine, except green tea, which has a low caffeine content; I drink it because it's high in antioxidants and has other healthy benefits.

I've already mentioned flavored carbonated sodas. Even when they are sugar- and caffeine-free, they have very little nutritional value. The main problem is that many people drink them instead of water or healthier beverages. Spritzers – fruit juices mixed with carbonated water – can make a healthy carbonated drink, however.

What about sports drinks? Basically, the average person doesn't need them. They were designed to replace the electrolytes lost by athletes or by others who participate in very strenuous exercise.

WATER, WATER, WATER -
AND OTHER BEVERAGES

That leaves fruit and vegetable juices. Virtually all of them are healthy.

Fresh-squeezed juices usually have the most nutrients, especially if some of the pulp is included. But many frozen and canned juices are nearly as beneficial, especially those with added calcium and vitamin C. It's important to check labels, however, for sugar, and especially for sodium, content.

The best route to take with beverages may be to drink a healthy variety throughout the day, especially water. This allows your body to realize the health benefits of a variety of sources of fluids.

CHAPTER 6
THE BEST FOODS AND WHY

The past few chapters have included the importance of eating right, specific food terms, and the attributes of vitamins, minerals, sodium and beverages. Here's a look at some of the all-around best foods, those that will help you the most to get healthy and stay healthy. The first section on the best foods list was culled mainly from a roster of healthy foods in a January 28, 2002, *Time* magazine article called "10 Foods That Pack A Wallop." The second section lists some other exceptionally healthy foods, including a few that might surprise you.

10 Top Foods

Blueberries – Blueberries were used by American Indians for their curative power. They're especially good at boosting the immune system and are the source of multiple beneficial nutrients – numerous antioxidants, vitamin C, folic acid, fiber and many others. In fact, a study comparing them with more than 40 other fruits and vegetables showed blueberries have the most antioxidants.

Broccoli – Broccoli is one of the best of the cruciferous vegetables, which, when eaten on a regular basis, have been shown to help reduce the risks of colon, breast and stomach cancer. It has few calories and no fat whatsoever. But it is not suggested you eat all you want at once, due to its effectiveness as a natural laxative. Broccoli is loaded with vitamin C, fiber, calcium and antioxidants. It also may help make some cancer-causing agents harmless before they have a chance to do any damage. That includes cancer-causing estrogen in women and those agents causing prostate cancer in men.

Garlic – In its long history, garlic has been credited with everything from healing sickness to warding off vampires. Today, there are very good indications garlic can help ward off heart disease. The strong sulfur-based substances in garlic, which are responsible for its pungent odor, can lower cholesterol and blood pressure, and possibly prevent blood clots. Garlic may also prevent or fight some cancers. There are indications it helps prevent or fight infection with its antibacterial, anti-parasite, antiviral and anti-fungal properties, and may even help get rid of nasal congestion. To get the most benefit from garlic, crush it before using.

Oats – Oats are another great source of fiber, which helps keep people regular. But eating unrefined oats or oatmeal often can also help lower cholesterol and may help lower blood pressure.

Salmon – Salmon is considered the best source of omega-3 of all the fatty fishes. Omega-3s have many healthy elements, including the ability to prevent platelets from becoming clumped and sticking to artery walls. Salmon helps lower triglyceride and LDL cholesterol, and may protect brain cells from Alzheimer's and age-related diseases.

Spinach – Another colorful, heart-healthy vegetable, spinach is low in calories and has no fat, so you can eat all you want. It's full of iron and folate that lower the amount of the amino acid homocystine in the bloodstream, which has been linked to heart problems. It also has two phytochemicals called lutein and zeaxanthin, believed to reduce the risk of age-related macular degeneration, which can cause blindness. Spinach is also the best source of vegetable protein and is high in calcium and vitamins A and C. It also has flavonoids and antioxidant properties that may block cancer-causing processes and substances.

Green and Black Tea – It's been known for some time that green tea is good for your health but black tea may be almost as good. Although processed differently, they come from the same kind of leaves. These teas have been known to prevent certain cancers, and they have much higher levels of antioxidants than even vitamin C.

Tomatoes – Tomatoes are a great source of lycopene, credited with being the most effective antioxidant to defuse free radicals. Lycopene in tomatoes is best released by cooking, but uncooked tomatoes (as well as cooked) are a good source of vitamin C.

Walnuts – While all nuts can help lower cholesterol, walnuts are the ones that do the best job. They are also probably the best source of plant-based omega-3, one of the "healthy" fats. It doesn't take more than a handful a day to get the full benefit – which is a good thing, because also like all nuts, walnuts are very high in calories. Walnuts have other nutrients that lower the risk of cardiovascular disease, not to mention the variety of other benefits attributed to omega-3s.

Wine – Red wine has strong antioxidants that can boost HDL (good) cholesterol levels when consumed in moderation and now there is evidence that white wine may do the same. However, while this works well in men, there are now concerns that a daily glass or two of wine may not have the same benefits for women. It is therefore suggested that women limit their consumption of wine to one glass daily; men a maximum of one or two glasses daily. However, most researchers and physicians advise against starting to drink wine for the health benefits if you don't drink it already.

Other Beneficial Foods

Apples – It's probably no surprise, but apples really can help keep the doctor away. Eating plenty of apples, including the peel, helps protect the lungs, and studies also indicate that apples are among the most effective fruits for reducing risks of developing serious disease. Apples also have a lot of the mineral boron, believed to reduce calcium loss and increase alertness. The average apple is low in calories and fat and has plenty of fiber, especially the kind called pectin, which is believed to lower cholesterol and regulate blood sugar.

Avocado – You may have heard avocados are high in fat. It's true, but it's mainly the good kind, unsaturated fat. They also have plenty of fiber and lots of vitamins C and B6. Half an avocado is about 150 calories and has about one-third of most people's daily requirement of folate, another heart-healthy element.

Chili Peppers – Yes, they're hot, but if your digestive tract can handle them, they may help you lose weight. They do this by suppressing appetite and increasing metabolism to burn up more calories. They're a great source of vitamins C and A – and they may even help clear up sinus congestion!

Cinnamon – Cinnamon has been found to help lower blood sugar, cholesterol and triglycerides and also to improve how insulin functions. A half-teaspoon of cinnamon daily provides these benefits. Use it instead of sugar or honey for seasoning and boil cinnamon sticks in water to make a zesty cup of tea.

Cocoa – Research findings reported in the December 2003 issue of the *Journal of Agricultural and Food Chemistry* have shown cocoa with no sugar or other added ingredients may be helpful in reducing heart disease. In fact, according to Dr. Chang Yon Lee, one of the scientists involved in the joint study between Cornell University and Seoul National University, it has more heart-healthy antioxidants per serving than some other heart-healthy beverages, including twice the amount in red wine, two or three times the amount in green tea, and four or five times the amount in black tea. Although chocolate, especially dark chocolate, has similar antioxidant properties, it is not really recommended for antioxidant use because of its high calories, saturated fat and sugar content.

Oranges – Citrus fruits have been shown to reduce the risks of a variety of health problems, and recent studies indicate oranges have a very high level of antioxidants, including more than 60 flavonoids with the ability to defend against tumors, blood clotting and inflammation. Oranges have fiber and folate to prevent damage from free radicals, strengthen the immune cells, and are a major source of vitamin C. New evidence has surfaced linking oranges and fresh-squeezed orange juice to a decreased risk of developing cataracts, certain kinds of anemia and high LDL cholesterol.

Peanut Butter – Peanut butter, that staple of our childhood days, really is good for you. A Harvard University study reported in the November 2002 issue of *The Journal of the American Medical Association* showed that women who ate peanut butter at least five times a week, or an equitable amount of peanuts, reduced their diabetes risk by 21 percent over women who didn't. It's also a good source of fiber, and its unsaturated fat can help keep fat and cholesterol out of the bloodstream. Like other nut-based foods, peanut butter has the amino acid arginine, believed to relax blood vessels, thus keeping blood pressure down. But check the labels. Most commercial peanut butters have hydrogenated vegetable oils and high sodium and sugar content. Natural peanut butter made solely from unsalted peanuts is a better choice.

Bell Peppers – Related to chili peppers, but much milder and sweeter, bell peppers have much to offer in the way of food benefits. They ripen only before they're picked, so once they're off the vine they are green, yellow or red. They are all a great source of vitamin C.

Prunes – When most people think of prunes or prune juice, they may think of a fruit used to relieve constipation. But prunes may do a lot more than that, especially for postmenopausal women. New research suggests prunes, which contain pectin fiber, may slow down the rise in cholesterol common in women after menopause. In addition, they may help eliminate the bone loss that occurs in osteoporosis that can lead to fractures, and they may aid in forming new bone.

Pumpkin – Pumpkins are very high in potassium, have substantial amounts of the antioxidants vitamin C and beta-carotene, and are also a good source of calcium and other vitamins and minerals. Pumpkinseed oil and pumpkin seeds are good sources of zinc and unsaturated fatty acids. They may also help you lose weight. According to a study by the United States Department of Agriculture (USDA), diets high in pumpkin as a source of fiber tended to curb appetite but had a high nutritional value for the amount of calories that were consumed. Study participants also absorbed fewer calories and less fat from their food. The government's 2005 dietary guidelines also tout pumpkinseeds as a good source of omega-3s.

Soy – Soy, a staple in most Asian diets, is another cholesterol-lowering food that many nutritionists now believe also offers several other benefits to the cardiovascular system. Soy comes in a variety of forms – from tofu to fortified milk. But use a low-sodium version of soy sauce, rather than the usual higher-sodium version. As an alternative to tofu, green soybeans, called edamame by the Japanese, are great for snacks.

Turmeric – Curcumin is the active ingredient in the spice turmeric and in results published in the September 2002 issue of the medical journal *Blood* was shown to suppress cancer cells and stop them from spreading. It was not recommended for patients undergoing chemotherapy, however. Other benefits of turmeric include easing arthritis and muscle pain, postoperative pain and swelling.

Watermelon – Like tomato, watermelon is a great source of the antioxidant lycopene, which has been shown to fight cancer, particularly in the prostate. Studies have suggested it may also keep plaque from building up in the arteries and offset damage caused by pollution, poor diet and aging – conditions that can lead to Alzheimer's and Parkinson's diseases and arthritis, in addition to cancers and heart disease.

Yogurt – Yogurt, the fat-free kind, has all sorts of healthy elements. It's a great source of calcium, providing 20 percent to 25 percent per serving of what most people need daily. Calcium can reduce the chance of fractures from osteoporosis as people grow older, may reduce the risk of colon polyps, and can even help people take off weight. Some yogurt contains live cultures of acidophilus, which makes it easier for some people to digest. A number of lower-fat yogurts do contain sugar products. To get the best results, try non-fat plain yogurt and mix it with fresh fruits. Fat-free yogurt also makes a good base for salad dressings and sauces.

More Good News About Healthy Foods

Research in recent years has indicated that what kinds of foods people eat may determine where excess fat is stored in the body. This is important because fat cells act differently from one another when stored in different parts of the body. In a body shape known as the pear shape, where most fat is stored around the hips and thighs, fat is not as metabolically active as when it's stored around the organs in the abdomen, that is, when people have an apple or round shape.

THE BEST FOODS AND WHY

The fat in the abdomen area is associated with serious health problems such as diabetes and hypertension. A study at Tufts University put participants on two diets with the same amount of calories, but from different food sources. A number of the people who ate more white bread, white rice and other refined foods than the participants on the different diet tended to add more fat around their waists, sometimes even when they didn't gain weight. Most of those on the diet that encompassed more whole grains and unrefined foods, however, did not add fat around the waist.

Healthiest Foods By Category

Fruit

Fruit	Amt.	Cal.	Carb.	Fats	Fiber	Vitamins
Apples	1 med.	73	19 gr.	0	10 gr.**	A, C
Avocado	1 large	369 *	13 gr.	37 gr.*	8 gr.	A, C
Blueberries	1 cup	81	21 gr.	0	4 gr.	A, C
Cantaloupe	1 cup	56	13 gr.	0	1 gr.	A
Oranges	1 med.	64	16 gr.	0	3 gr.	A, C
Papayas	1 cup	54	14 gr.	0	4 gr.	A, C
Prunes	5 dried	100	26 gr.	0	3 gr. **	A
Raspberries	1 cup	60	11 gr.	1 gr.	8 gr.	A, C
Watermelon	1 cup	154	35 gr.	2 gr.	2 gr.	A, C

The food elements listed here include only those most important in fruits. Cholesterol for example, is not shown because fruits have none. Sodium is not listed because most fruits have very little.

Abbreviations used:
   Gr. = grams

   * Although avocados are high in calories and fat, the fat is mainly healthy unsaturated fat, with only 6 grams of saturated fat per large avocado.
  ** Apples contain pectin fiber, believed to lower cholesterol and regulate blood sugar. So do prunes.

THE BEST FOODS AND WHY

Healthiest Foods By Category

Vegetables

Vegetable	Amt.	Cal.	Carb.	Fats	Fiber	Vitamins
Bell peppers*	1 large	20	5 gr.	0	1 gr.	A, C
Broccoli	1 cup	44	12 gr.	0	5 gr.	A, C
Cabbage	1 cup	35	8 gr.	0	4 gr.	A, C
Chili peppers	1 cup	18	4 gr.	7 gr.	1 gr.	A, C
Garlic	1/4 cup	42	9 gr.	0	2 gr.	Low
Pumpkin	1 cup	49	12 gr.	0	4 gr.	A, C
Spinach	1 cup	41	7 gr.	0	4 gr.	A, C
Tomatoes	1 medium	42	6 gr.	0	2 gr.	A, C

The food elements listed here include only those most important in vegetables. Cholesterol, for example, is not shown because vegetables have none. Sodium is no listed because most vegetables have very little.

Abbreviations used:
  gr. = grams

* This is for orange & red peppers. Green peppers have same but in lesser amounts.

61

Healthiest Foods By Category

Meats, Poultry and Fish

Food	Amt.	Cal.	Sodium	Fats	Chol.	Protein
Round steak	3 oz. *	153	52 mg.	4 gr.	71 mg.	27 gr.
Chicken	3 oz. **	138	59 mg.	3.5 gr.	65 mg.	27 gr.
Turkey	3 oz. ***	119	48 mg.	1 gr.	73 mg.	26 gr.
Flounder	3 oz.	97	77 mg.	1 gr.	51 mg.	20 gr.
Salmon	3 oz.	155	22 mg.	7 gr. ****	60 mg.	22 gr.
Salmon (Canned)	3 oz.	118	64 mg.	5 gr.	47 mg.	17 gr.

The food elements listed here include only those most important in meats, poultry, fish and dairy.

Abbreviations used:
> Gr. = grams
> Mg. = milligrams

* Round steak is the leanest of beef cuts; this is based on trimmed and broiled choice beef
** Skinned, boned and poached chicken breast
*** Roasted turkey breast
**** Only 1 gram of fat is saturated, the rest includes omega 3 oils, of which salmon has the highest amount of any fish

Healthiest Foods By Category
Dairy Products

Food	Amt.	Cal.	Fats	Sat. Fat	Chol.	Calcium
Skim milk	1 cup *	90	0.5 gr.	4	5 mg.	312 mg.
2% fat milk	1 cup *	130	5 gr.	3 gr.	20 mg.	300 mg.
FF half & half	1 cup	158	0	0	0	16 mg.
FF plain yogurt	1 cup	132	0	0	4 mg.	475 mg.
FF cottage cheese	1 cup	160	0	0	0	160 mg.
FF cheddar	1 oz.	50	0	0	0	123 mg.
FF cream cheese	2 Tbsp.	30	0	0	0	minimal
Smart Balance Omega Plus Buttery Spread **	1 Tbsp.	80	2.5 gr.	2.5 gr.	0	minimal

The food elements listed here include only those most important in dairy products

Abbreviations used:

      Chol. = cholesterol   mg. = milligrams
      gr. = grams   Sat. Fat = saturated fat
      FF = fat free

  * 1 cup = 8 oz.
 ** not a dairy product, shown only as an example of butter substitute;
     contains no trans fat

CHAPTER 7

THE WORST FOODS AND WHY

Foods to Avoid or Consume in Small Amounts

Refined grains – This includes white rice, white bread, white pasta and other products made with white flour. Refining removes most of the nutrients. While these foods are enriched with certain nutrients as required by federal law, not all the missing nutrients are necessarily put back in. In addition, the refining process deletes most of the fiber and converts these products into simple sugars.

This can mean that for those who have normal blood sugar levels and aren't diabetic, instead of digesting the sugar content slowly as it does with many non-refined carbohydrates, the body digests it very quickly. Any sugar not used by the body may trigger the pancreas to overreact and release insulin.

This may cause the body to store sugar as fat, and it may cause the insulin, in turn, to drop blood sugar levels too low, possibly triggering hunger and faintness. If this happens too often, the body may stop responding properly to insulin, possibly triggering Type 2 diabetes.

Most other white foods – This includes white potatoes, which can trigger the same up-and-down sugar reaction as refined grains, and coconut, which is full of saturated fat. Follow this "no-white" rule in your diet, with the exception of garlic, onion and cauliflower.

Foods containing trans fat – This includes vegetable shortenings, stick margarine and other foods that have been made with partially hydrogenated vegetable oils, even from healthy oils like soybean or olive oils. Once hydrogenated, these oils contain trans fatty acids, and are no longer healthy. Check the ingredients list on labels for partially hydrogenated oils, the "hidden" trans fat.

However, sometimes a label advertises that a product has no trans fat but still shows partially hydrogenated vegetable oil on the ingredients list. This seems confusing, but the government allows it if the amount of partially hydrogenated oils is less than 0.05 percent. This probably should not be of too much concern as long as helpings are infrequent, portions are moderate and the nutrients in the product are beneficial.

Most fast food – Hamburgers, fried chicken, french fries, onion rings, etc. are on this list. They have too much saturated fat and often trans fat. Even the buns aren't healthy, as most are made with refined flours and unhealthy fats. The salad dressings used may have trans fat, saturated fat, sugar and/or sodium. Ask for no-fat dressings with no added sugar, Italian dressing with an oil base instead of cream, or oil and vinegar.

Unhealthy snacks – These include most cookies, potato chips, crackers and other snacks that are fried. These have too much saturated fat and/or trans fat and are very high in sodium and/or sugar.

Many organic packaged foods – Organic foods may be healthy for the environment but not always healthy for you. Check nutrition labels for calorie count and content to determine whether any of the following have been added: high sodium, saturated fat, trans fat, and/or high sugar.

Certain condiments – Although usually used in small amounts, many condiments such as regular ketchup and mustard are high in sodium and/or sugar. Instead choose low-sodium soy sauce, low-sugar, lower-sodium ketchup, and Dijon mustard.

Fatty red meats, fried poultry and fish, and poultry skin – This includes many beef products, like regular hamburger, and marbled beef such as steaks; and fried chicken, especially when the skin has not been removed, and which usually has been cooked in unhealthy fats. Avoid fried fish and other fried seafood also.

Certain cereals – Many cereals, while enriched, are made from refined grains and often have high sugar/sodium content and low fiber. Check ingredients list for refined flour; high sugar, including honey and molasses; and/or sodium.

THE WORST FOODS AND WHY

Certain desserts – These include processed and commercially baked cakes, pies and cookies, as well as baked goods you might make yourself with high sugar content (including molasses, honey, brown sugar, etc.); saturated fats (butter); shortenings such as solid margarine (trans fat); and even salt, and ice cream. When eating these desserts, try taking just a few bites. When possible, try the non-fat, non-sugar desserts instead.

CHAPTER 8

A NEW LOOK
AT THE FOOD GUIDE PYRAMID

Food Guide Pyramids

The best-known food guide pyramid is the U.S. Department of Agriculture (USDA) pyramid created in 1992. We've all seen it hundreds of times – it's everywhere. It is a good idea because people can look at it and easily tell which foods should be eaten sparingly and which should take up a larger portion of their diet. The only problem is that it was out of date even when it was released, and it's not very scientifically based.

Although it was created by the government ostensibly as a guideline to healthier eating for Americans, heavy lobbying from the agriculture, beef, dairy and other food industries influenced its make-up. So it isn't necessarily a very good guide to the most healthful way to eat.

Over the years, however, the concept of a healthy eating pyramid has been more widely accepted, and now there are numerous interpretations of it. I have even made one of my own, which you'll see later in this chapter.

A new Food Guide Pyramid from the USDA should take in the government's latest Nutrition Guidelines for Americans, which have some healthier elements.* But first, let's take a look at the current USDA pyramid and examine each segment:

Bread, cereal, rice and pasta – These are grouped together, with six to 11 servings recommended daily. At the time the pyramid was created, all fats were considered unhealthy, which today we know is not true. Emphasis was placed instead on carbohydrates. We now know not all grains are healthy. They definitely should play a significant role in our diets, but whole grains and other complex carbohydrates need to be emphasized. Grouping all grains together does not properly indicate that refined grains and other "white" foods should be avoided.

This is one of the main problems with the USDA pyramid – that both healthy and unhealthy foods are grouped together. For example,

Food Guide Pyramid
A Guide to Daily Food Choices

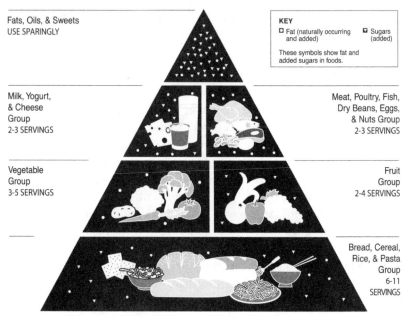

Fats, Oils, & Sweets
USE SPARINGLY

KEY
◻ Fat (naturally occurring   🔲 Sugars
   and added)   (added)

These symbols show fat and
added sugars in foods.

Milk, Yogurt,
& Cheese
Group
2-3 SERVINGS

Meat, Poultry, Fish,
Dry Beans, Eggs,
& Nuts Group
2-3 SERVINGS

Vegetable
Group
3-5 SERVINGS

Fruit
Group
2-4 SERVINGS

Bread, Cereal,
Rice, & Pasta
Group
6-11
SERVINGS

Source: U.S. Department of Agriculture/U.S. Department of Health and Human Services

there is nothing on it to indicate there are both healthy and unhealthy fats. This implies all fats are alike, so people are not really getting all the correct information they need to eat properly.

In addition, the USDA grouped all fats and oils with desserts, with the caution to "use sparingly." While saturated fats and trans fat – the "unhealthy" fats – should be avoided, healthy unsaturated fats (monounsaturated fats and polyunsaturated fats, including omega-3s) should be included and clearly indicated on the food guide pyramid.

Vegetables – The government pyramid shows three to five servings. Vegetables are very important in a healthy diet, but there are exceptions, such as white potatoes that can act in the body like simple sugars and should be excluded. This section should focus on healthy vegetables like

68

broccoli and cauliflower, green leafy vegetables like spinach, and brightly colored vegetables such as tomatoes. Although technically tomatoes are fruits, the general public seems to put them in the vegetable bin.

Fruits – These are certainly wonderful for you, but I believe three to five servings daily are more appropriate than the two to four shown on the USDA pyramid.

Milk, yogurt and cheese – Two to three servings daily are recommended in this category. I don't have a problem with this amount of dairy products, but whole milk, cheese and yogurt have a lot of saturated fat. This food grouping should indicate non-fat or low-fat dairy foods only.

Meat, poultry, eggs, fish and nuts – These foods are all grouped together at two to three servings daily. I think they should be grouped separately as follows:

- Lean meats, rather than marbled meats.
- Skinless white meat chicken and turkey, usually the breast.
- Fish that supply a lot of healthy omega-3 fats, such as salmon.
- Nuts, which are also great sources of healthy fats, especially walnuts and almonds.
- Egg whites and egg substitutes.

Fats, oils and sweets – "Use sparingly," the USDA pyramid says. But unhealthy fats and oils like saturated fat, palm and coconut oils, and partially hydrogenated vegetable oils (trans fat) should be excluded. Instead, the pyramid should show only healthy unsaturated fats, like monounsaturated and polyunsaturated fats, including omega-3s. Healthy sweets that are non-fat and sugar-free are fine but should not be grouped with fats and oils.

The government's pyramid is based on the Dietary Guidelines for Americans. These are updated every five years by a panel of nutrition experts from a variety of backgrounds, and the 2005 guidelines are the most recent. It's important to recognize the financial and nutritional impact of these dietary guidelines, which set the standards for all federal

A NEW LOOK
AT THE FOOD GUIDE PYRAMID

nutrition programs, such as school lunch programs, outside-school-hours programs, and nutrition assistance to low-income families. The guidelines also advise Americans on what foods are the most nutritious and healthiest to eat. Consequently, the panel of experts can be subject to a lot of pressure from special interest groups in the country's multibillion-dollar food industry.

The Seretean Pyramid

After years of studying, learning and practicing good nutrition, I've come up with a food guide pyramid I think more accurately reflects how people should eat to reap the most health benefits from their diets.

The Seretean Pyramid

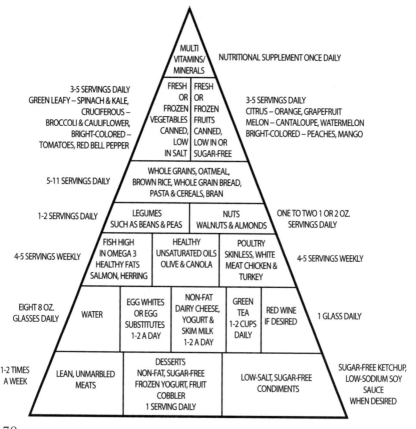

A NEW LOOK
AT THE FOOD GUIDE PYRAMID

It's unbiased because it wasn't influenced by any outside interests but only by the beliefs, backed by scientific research, of a senior citizen trying to live a healthy lifestyle.

As you can see, this pyramid is quite different than the USDA's. For example, although vitamin and mineral supplements aren't food, many physicians advise their patients to take a daily multi-vitamin/multi-mineral supplement to cover any shortcomings in the diet as a kind of insurance policy for good health. So these are included on the pyramid.

Water, which also is not a food but is so important to good health, is also included. The old standard of drinking eight 8-ounce glasses daily still stands.

What I've tried to do is include only what people should eat in each food group, give some of the examples of each when applicable, and suggest how many portions should be eaten daily. As I suggested earlier when reviewing the USDA pyramid, the healthiest kinds of vegetables are the ones I've mentioned; for example, those that are brightly colored. The fruit segment has been devised in a similar manner.

The only grains included are whole grains, and I've given several examples. No refined, processed grains are mentioned. I think five to 11 servings daily, the same amount recommended on the USDA pyramid, is good advice.

Nuts have their own category and so do legumes, each with a few examples of the best kinds. Several servings daily are fine for legumes, but nuts should be eaten in moderation. Although they are very good for you, they're high in calories.

Poultry, lean meats and fish also are in separate categories. They're all considered meat, but each is different. For example, poultry is strictly defined as skinless white meat with no mention of the darker, fattier parts like drumsticks. And it should be served grilled, baked or broiled, not fried, in up to five servings a week. Meats are OK at one to two servings weekly, but lean meat is emphasized. Fish, mainly those high in omega-3 polyunsaturated fats, are emphasized at four to five servings a week. Other sources of healthy unsaturated oils are in a category by themselves, with examples given.

I've devoted a little space to condiments because most of them have either high sugar or high-sodium content, and sometimes both. However, there are a number of products available with no salt and sugar added.

A NEW LOOK
AT THE FOOD GUIDE PYRAMID

A few good examples, such as no-sodium, sugar-free ketchup, are shown on the pyramid.

Green tea is in a separate category, as is wine. Both can contribute to good health, but red wine should be taken in moderation, hence the recommended amount of one glass daily – but only if desired, since people who don't ordinarily drink alcohol are usually advised not to start.

Non-fat dairy products are the only kind I recommend, at one or two servings a day. The Seretean Pyramid suggests egg whites or egg substitutes rather than whole eggs.

Desserts have not been forgotten, but I suggest sugar-free, non-fat treats and have recommended a couple that are both healthy and tasty choices.

As you can see, this pyramid focuses on healthy foods, beverages and nutrients. Everything on it is good for you. It also gives you easily understood information and is much more specific and healthier than the USDA Food Guide Pyramid.

It is also important to let you know I don't follow these suggested food and portion guidelines anywhere close to 100 percent of the time, although I try to as much as possible. The more you can adhere to this food guide pyramid, however, the greater the positive impact on your health. Any percentage of it that you adopt is a plus.

* An updated food guide pyramid, MyPyramid, was released by the government in 2005. As it was at the time of publication of this book, however, it could not be included or addressed.

CHAPTER 9

HOW TO READ A FOOD LABEL

The nutrition labeling required by the government for many foods is a great source of information for people who are trying to eat in the most healthful way possible.

Labeling is required on the majority of pre-packaged foods – crackers, cookies, dairy products, juices, frozen foods and others. There are a few exceptions, however. These include fresh vegetables and fruits, food served for immediate consumption, such as airline meals; ready-to-eat foods prepared on site, including candy or bakery items; foods for medical patients; plain coffee and tea; some spices; and foods that contain no significant amounts of nutrients.

However, some nutrition information is available for a number of raw foods on a voluntary basis from the retailer. This voluntary labeling includes the 20 most frequently eaten raw vegetables, fruit and fish, and the 45 best-selling cuts of meat. While not required, the majority of retailers do supply some nutrition information for most of these products. They must adhere, however, to strict regulations as to how this information may be used.

Most of us are at least somewhat familiar with the Nutrition Facts panel on food packaging, but there is additional information on the food package that can help us make good food choices. These are shown on the ingredients list, and in some instances, show food claims, which are terms describing the foods. These include such terms as "fat-free," "low-sodium," and "fresh."

The Nutrition Facts Panel

Some parts of the Nutrition Facts panel seem easy to understand, such as the sodium or saturated-fat content. Others seem more difficult – what the heck is a Daily Value anyway? But once you understand what the information means and become familiar with it, you can tell at a glance what you need to know. Here's a description of the components and how the information should be used. Some pieces of information are required on the Nutrition Facts panel and some that aren't required are allowed if the manufacturer wishes to include them.

This information is mandatory:

Total calories
Calories from fat
Total fat
Saturated fat
Cholesterol
Sodium
Total carbohydrate
Dietary fiber
Sugars
Sugar alcohols
 (sugar substitutes such as sorbitol)
Protein
Vitamin A
Vitamin C
Calcium
Iron

This information is voluntary:

Calories from saturated fat
Polyunsaturated fat
Monounsaturated fat
Potassium
Soluble fiber
Insoluble fiber
Other carbohydrates
% of vitamin A present as beta carotene
Other essential vitamins and minerals
Trans fat (will be required)

These required and optional food components are the only ones allowed on a Nutrition Facts panel or table. Information about calories from polyunsaturated fats or from carbohydrates, for example, doesn't appear in the panel. Furthermore, if a claim is made about any optional components, or if the food is either fortified or enriched, that information is required on the label.

When the Nutrition Facts panel was created, it reflected the health concerns of the time. These elements had to appear on the panel in the order of what was considered their priority.

Changes for the Nutrition Facts panel are now under consideration because healthy eating priorities have changed quite a bit since the format was drawn up.

In addition, the committees determining dietary guidelines for nutrients have changed some of the daily recommended amounts of certain nutrients, such as sodium, which will appear on the Nutrition Facts panel in the next few years.

Now, let's get down to business. Here's what you'll find on the panel:

HOW TO READ A FOOD LABEL

Serving size – The panel must use simple everyday terms of measurement such as slice, cup or tablespoon to describe the size of the serving and must also state the serving size in grams or milligrams in parentheses. But bear in mind that, although the Food and Drug Administration (FDA) says the serving size is based on what people actually eat, many of you will find the serving sizes much smaller than the portion you would usually consume.

Servings per container – This must state how many servings of the indicated size are included in the package.

Calories – It must next show the number of calories in a serving and how many of those calories come from fat.

Nutrients and percentage of Daily Value – The next part of the panel lists the amounts of several important nutrients along with their percentage of the Daily Value (DV). These nutrients are those that are sources of energy (calories), and include total fat, saturated fat, total carbohydrate including dietary fiber, and protein. The percentage of the Daily Value is also listed for cholesterol, sodium and sometimes potassium, all of which don't have calories.

The DV is a term of reference and, as you can see by the footnote on the panel, is based on a diet of 2,000 calories daily. It also states that your DV may be higher or lower depending on your calorie needs.

The Daily Value is the total recommended daily amount of each nutrient, which adds up to 100 percent for each element listed. The percentage of the Daily Value is simply how much a serving of the particular food supplies of the recommended amount of a specific nutrient. For example, a slice (one serving) of whole-wheat bread may have 2 grams of dietary fiber, which supplies 8 percent of the suggested amount needed by people taking in 2,000 calories a day. The implication is that people on a 2,000-calorie diet should get 92 percent of their recommended amount of dietary fiber from other sources.

The total recommended Daily Values in percentages of the total calories taken in are:

- Fat based on 30 percent or less of calories.
- Saturated fat based on 10 percent or less of calories.

- Carbohydrate based on 60 percent or less of calories.
- Protein based on 10 percent or less of calories.
- Fiber based on 11.5 grams of dietary fiber per 1,000 calories.

For some reason, however, these aren't shown on the Nutrition Facts panel or other parts of the food label – which I believe is an oversight.

Under total carbohydrate, you will notice it's broken into at least two listings – dietary fiber and sugar, which are mandatory. Other forms of carbohydrate may be listed as well. You can also see that the amount of sugar is listed but does not have a percentage of Daily Value. Neither does protein. However, the vitamins and minerals shown have the percentage of Daily Value listed but not the amounts.

Finally at the bottom, there is a listing of the maximum recommended amount of certain nutrients that are of concern to public health for a 2,000-calorie diet. These include total fat, saturated fat, cholesterol, sodium, total carbohydrate and dietary fiber, and may include maximum recommended amounts for a 2,500-calorie diet as well. Some panels may also list the amount of calories per gram for fat, carbohydrate and protein.

To aid you in your search to find the healthiest foods, take a look at the graphic from the FDA showing a typical Nutrition Facts panel, along with simple explanations for each element. Not all panels look alike; they may have a different configuration because of the size and shape of the packaging. While some abbreviations are allowed when there are size constraints, all Nutrition Facts panels must have the same mandatory information.

The Ingredients List

There must also be a listing of ingredients on all food labels, unless there is only one ingredient, such as peanuts. Most food manufacturers, however, will include the single ingredient on the food label anyway.

The ingredients list doesn't give you the precise amount of each ingredient. However, ingredients must be listed in descending order of the amount by weight the food contains. For example, if whole-wheat flour is the first ingredient listed, followed by refined wheat flour, and then by water, you know there is more whole-wheat flour in the product than refined flour, and more of both whole wheat and refined flour than water.

A. How much there is in a serving size, with the amount of grams in a serving shown in parenthesis, & how many servings are in the container

B. How many calories there are in a serving & how many calories in a serving come from fat

C. The total fat in a serving, & of this, how much of the fat is saturated

D. The % of the Daily Value (DV) of various nutrients – that is, the percentage of that nutrient in each serving, based on the total amount (100 percent) recommended daily for people who want to take in 2,000 calories a day

E. Amt. of cholesterol & % DV

F. Amt. of sodium & % DV

G. Total carbohydrate & % DV

H. Additional information about the kind of carbohydrate in a serving -- here, the amount of Dietary Fiber & % DV

I. More information about the kind of carbohydrate in a serving -- here, the amount of sugars, but no information on the % DV

J. Amount of protein in a serving but again no information about what percentage there is based on Daily Value

K. % DV of vitamins A & C, calcium & iron

L. Footnote – self-explanatory

M. Recommendations on the maximum amount of certain nutrients a person on a 2,000-calorie diet should have every day. Also, voluntary information about the maximum amount suggested for a 2,500-calorie diet.

N. Voluntary information about number of calories per gram of certain nutrients

Nutrition Facts

Serving Size 1 piece (219g)
Servings Per Container 6

Amount Per Serving

Calories 520   Calories from Fat 240

% Daily Value*

Total Fat 27g	**41%**
Saturated Fat 12g	**61%**
Cholesterol 255mg	**86%**
Sodium 1110mg	**46%**
Total Carbohydrate 29g	**10%**
Dietary Fiber 1g	**5%**
Sugars 1g	
Protein 39g	

Vitamin A 20%	•	Vitamin C 4%
Calcium 15%	•	Iron 25%

*Percent Daily Values are based on a 2,000 calorie diet. Your daily values may be higher or lower depending on your calorie needs:

	Calories:	2,000	2,500
Total Fat	Less than	65g	80g
Saturated Fat	Less than	20g	25g
Cholesterol	Less than	300mg	300mg
Sodium	Less than	2,400mg	2,400mg
Total Carbohydrate		300g	375g
Dietary Fiber		25g	30g

Calories per gram:
Fat 9 • Carbohydrate 4 • Protein 4

In addition, the ingredients list can be helpful to the knowledgeable consumer in several other ways. It can reveal whether there are "hidden" ingredients that aren't shown or counted on the Nutrition Facts panel. For example, there are several allergens that could be included on the ingredients list but not necessarily in a form most people would recognize. Some of these include *whey* and *caseinate* from milk; *albumin, livetin* and *ovalbumin* from eggs; and *semolina* and *spelt* from wheat.

Food Claims

Food Nutrient Claims

There are a lot of these, but a working knowledge of what many of them mean can help you choose the healthiest foods. Government regulations determine what terms can be used to describe the levels of nutrients in food and how they can be used. Here is a list of some of the more important ones to know for healthy eating:

Free – Product does not contain, or contains an insignificant amount of, fat, saturated fat, cholesterol, sodium, sugars or calories, or a combination of one or more of these. Calorie free means less than 5 calories per serving; sugar-free and fat-free both mean less than 0.5 grams per serving. Synonyms include "without," "no," "zero" and for fat-free milk, "skim."

Low – Used when foods can be eaten often without going over the government's dietary guidelines for fat, saturated fat, cholesterol, sodium and calories, or a combination of two or more of these. The following amounts are used:

- **Low fat** – 3 grams or less per serving
- **Low saturated fat** – 1 gram or less per serving
- **Low sodium** – 140 mg. or less per serving
- **Very low sodium** – 35 mg. or less per serving
- **Low cholesterol** – 20 mg. or less and 2 grams or less of saturated fat per serving
- **Low calorie** – 40 calories or less per serving

HOW TO READ A FOOD LABEL

Synonyms for low include "little," "few," "low source of" and "containing a small amount of."

Lean and Extra Lean – Can be used to describe the fat content of meat, poultry, seafood and game meats. "Lean" means less than 10 grams of total fat, 4.5 grams or less of saturated fat, and less than 95 mg. of cholesterol per serving and per 100 grams. "Extra lean" means less than 5 grams of total fat, less than 2 grams saturated fat, and less than 95 mg. of cholesterol per serving and per 100 grams.

High – Can be used if a serving of the food has 20 percent or more of the DV for a particular nutrient, calcium, for example.

Good source of – Means one serving contains 10 to 19 percent of DV for a particular nutrient.

Reduced – Nutritionally altered product that has at least 25 percent less of a nutrient, such as fat or calories, than the regular product or reference product. This term can't be used if the regular or reference product already meets the requirement for a "low" claim.

Less or fewer – Means a food, whether altered or not, has 25 percent less of a nutrient or calories than a reference food, which in many cases doesn't have to be the same kind of food. For example, a manufacturer is allowed to say its pretzels have 25 percent less fat than potato chips.

Light – Means one of two things:

1) A product that has one-third fewer calories or half the fat of the reference food. If the reference food has 50 percent or more of its calories from fat, then the reduction has to be 50 percent of *that* fat.

2) That the sodium content of a low-calorie, low-fat food has been reduced by at least 50 percent.

"Light" can also be used to describe properties such as texture and color, like light brown sugar or "light and fluffy," as long as the label explains the meaning. Also, as long as they aren't misleading, alternative spellings and their synonyms of these descriptive claims, such as "hi" or "lite," are allowed.

Here are a couple more bits of information from the FDA that may be of interest to the healthy eater:

Percent fat-free – Means food must be very low in fat or fat-free and has to accurately reflect the amount of fat in 100 grams of the food. So if a food has 5 grams of fat per 100 grams of the food, it may say it is 95 percent fat-free.

Implied – Prohibited if it wrongfully implies it has or does not have a meaningful level of a nutrient. A product claiming to be made with an ingredient that is a source of fiber – such as "made with whole-wheat flour" – isn't allowed unless it contains enough of that ingredient to meet the definition of "a good source of fiber." A claim that a food has "no tropical oils" is allowed but only on foods that are low in saturated fats because consumers nowadays rightfully equate tropical oils – basically coconut, palm and palm kernel oils – with high saturated fat.

Health Claims

Food claims concerning health can generate a lot of confusion and possibly misinformation. Part of this has to do with the way the government allows food manufacturers to label food product claims. It isn't necessarily consistent. For example, Sunsweet claims its prunes, like other fibrous foods, may help reduce the risk of heart disease and some cancers. This is OK because claims about specific diseases are pretty reliable usually, based either on "significant scientific agreement" about the evidence or on an "authoritative statement" by a government scientific panel.

On the other hand, claims that a particular product positively affects a bodily structure, such as bones, or function, such as urinary tract health, should be scrutinized because they don't have to be reviewed by the FDA. Food producers are required to supply evidence to support the claim only if the FDA challenges it. Unlike nutritional supplements, which by law have to include a disclaimer on the label, food products don't require any mention whatsoever on the packaging that the FDA has not reviewed the claims about them.

Sometimes claims are accurate but don't tell the whole story. Claims that a food is a good source of fiber, for example, may neglect to mention other information about the product, such as perhaps a high sugar or salt content. That's why it is so important consumers not pay too much attention to food health claims but instead carefully read both the Nutrition Facts panel and the ingredients list. This label information, based on government standards, is required by law to be accurate.

And while many nutritional health claims are justified, they usually apply to other foods in the same category as well, not to just that particular food or brand.

The FDA has actually authorized only 10 health claims for food. Some of these include: calcium as reducing the risk for osteoporosis, low sodium as reducing the risk of high blood pressure, and a diet low in sugar as helping to prevent tooth decay.

In addition, the American Heart Association has a program to indicate foods that are considered heart healthy. Foods that meet these AHA standards are allowed to display what's known as a "heart check" mark on the label. This does not cover a number of foods, however, that most scientists and researchers consider "heart healthy."

Also, bear in mind that no matter how accurate the nutrition claim may be, it can't in itself create good health. You need an overall healthy lifestyle to do that.

Putting It All Together

So now you have a plethora of information about nutrition labeling. How can you possibly remember it all? The answer, of course, is that you can't. The purpose of presenting it is to help you read food labels, to understand what they mean and how they work to avoid confusion, so you can interpret them correctly. So you might want to make note of those components that seem to be the most relevant for you to make healthy food choices. Then you can practice reading and assessing food labels by examining products that are already in your home.

The first place to start making healthy food choices is at the supermarket. Later in this book I'll address how to shop healthy once you're there. Meanwhile, let's do a mental test run as if you were already at a grocery store.

- You probably wouldn't pay much attention to food health claims but would actually be keeping an eye out for nutrient claims such as "fat-free" or "sugar-free."

- You would go straight to the Nutrition Facts panel on the label to see how much one serving of each product contains of fiber, calories, unsaturated fat, saturated fat and trans fat if it's included; carbohydrates, including dietary fiber, sugars and possibly others; and protein, vitamins and minerals.

- You'd take a good look at the serving size, being realistic about how many of the quoted serving sizes it would take to make up an actual serving for you. It could be several.

- You would read the list of ingredients, checking to make sure the product contained no hydrogenated vegetable oils or allergens, if you are allergic to certain foods.

This information would give you a truer picture of the food and help you assess whether you think it's a healthy choice for you.

So, let's take a look at an imaginary food label, such as the labeling on a "lite" salad dressing. The label says it's a reduced-calorie dressing with 4.5 grams of fat per serving, compared with 9 grams of fat in a serving of the manufacturer's regular salad dressing. In addition, it says there are 80 calories per serving compared with 110 calories in the regular salad dressing.

The Nutrition Facts panel shows 40 of those 80 calories are from fat and that the 4.5 grams of total fat is 7 percent of the DV for a 2,000-calorie diet. The product also contains no saturated fat or cholesterol, 120 mg. of sodium (5 percent of the DV) and a total carbohydrate of 10 grams, equivalent to about 3 percent DV. There is no fiber under the carbohydrate listing but there are 9 grams of sugar. There is also no vitamin A or C or any calcium or iron.

HOW TO READ A FOOD LABEL

Here is the list of ingredients: Sugar, water, vinegar, canola oil, onions, onion powder, modified food starch, salt, spices, potassium sorbate and calcium disodium EDTA as preservatives, natural flavor, and xanthan gum.

We see that sugar is first, so there has to be more sugar than any other ingredient. We can pretty well assume there isn't too much, however, because only 9 of the 10 grams of carbohydrate are sugar.

But now is a good time to make an assessment of the sugar in the salad dressing. Try to think of it this way: how much of your daily carbohydrate intake do you want to be simple sugars rather than complex carbohydrates that include fiber? If you aren't going to be eating a lot of sugar elsewhere in your diet, this amount may be insignificant when weighed against the benefits of reduced fat and calories. If you eat a lot of salad daily, however, and you like it slathered with salad dressing – even a reduced-fat one – you will be having much more than the two tablespoons considered a serving. So the sugar could really start to add up.

We don't know exactly how much canola oil the product contains, but we do know it's a healthy fat, with no trans fat hidden because there is no partially hydrogenated oil. There are also spices and sodium, which we already know is low from the Nutrition Facts panel. Other ingredients are xanthan gum and modified food starch, which are used as thickeners and emulsifiers; and preservatives and natural flavor, which seem simple enough and don't have any nutritional value. So it is pretty safe to assume we have the information we need and that, in fact, in reasonable amounts, the salad dressing seems to be a pretty healthy product.

However, this would be the time to do comparisons with other salad dressings. Therefore, you could also check out the fat-free varieties. Chances are you would find even less fat, so taking into consideration all the other nutrient information available, you could determine which is healthiest for you.

I don't really suggest adding up percentages or counting calories on a regular basis. First, it's way too much work. You can essentially keep your calories down by eating healthy foods in moderate amounts.

Secondly, the 2,000-calorie daily diet is an arbitrary figure. It's meant to be a reference point, and your caloric needs may be more or less depending on your age, your gender, your state of health and your activity level. You might want to check with your doctor about your calorie needs. And third, imagine how much work it would be to try to adjust up or down from a 2,000-calorie diet what your daily allowances should be depending on how many calories you've been advised to take in.

Food labeling is an excellent concept designed to help us figure out the best ways to eat. Coupled with knowledge about healthy eating, they are two of our best chances to learn to make good food choices.

The source for the majority of the information in this chapter is the FDA. But it isn't possible here to include everything about food labels. For more information about the agency and more detailed information about food labeling, go to the following website: www.cfsan.fda.gov/label.html. Or contact the FDA toll free at 1-888-INFO-FDA (1-888-463-6322). For detailed information about using the Nutrition Facts panel, go to http://vm.cfsan.fda.gov/~dms/foodlab.html.

CHAPTER 10

STAPLES, STORE LIST
AND KITCHEN EQUIPMENT

Before heading to the supermarket, you'll want to make a grocery list that will help you shop healthy so you can eat healthy. Be sure to keep certain staples on hand that will make it easier to eat in the healthiest way possible. These staples will provide most of what you need to create and cook healthy recipes, including those listed at the back of the book. You'll also want to purchase fresh foods, along with some frozen and packaged foods. Some suggestions about kitchen equipment that can be useful for preparing food are also included in this chapter.

Staples

Every household has its own list of staples, those items that are used for many purposes and are especially good to have in a pinch. The products suggested here include those that can be used to prepare or cook a variety of healthy meals and snacks. Among them are:

Healthy unsaturated oils – such as olive, canola and sesame oils. Virgin olive oil is the best of its kind because it has the most pungent taste. Canola is good because it adds little taste, while sesame provides an interesting flavor.

Various cooking sprays – such as olive, canola, butter-flavored and others. These have virtually no calories. You can also make your own flavored cooking spray with olive oil, Italian seasonings and a few herbs. Let them blend together for a few days, then empty into a spray container for tasty results.

Balsamic and white vinegars – for more variety, include red or white wine vinegar and/or rice wine vinegar.

Whole-wheat pita bread – this can be frozen until needed and used in a variety of ways.

Fat-free dairy products – plain yogurt, yogurt cheese, various kinds of cottage cheese, skim milk. If you can't find these, choose low-fat products.

Whole-grain cereals, bread and pasta – look for 100 percent whole-wheat (stone ground is best) or other whole-grain products. If not 100 percent, check the labels to make sure products proclaiming whole wheat or other whole grains list whole grain as the first ingredient. Many breads can be frozen until needed without much loss of flavor or freshness.

Blended-grain products – partially whole grain (usually wheat) with some refined flour are good choices when people are just beginning to add fiber to their diets.

Other whole grains – brown rice, wild rice, oats, brown basmati rice, or couscous. Don't buy the instant kinds, however, as nutrients can be lost in the processing.

Plain oatmeal – the kind you have to cook for a while. I recommend McCann's.

Artificial sweetener – such as Splenda, the brand name for sucralose.

Canned fish, unsalted or with low sodium if possible – sardines, salmon and white tuna.

Low-fat Miracle Whip – to use in place of mayonnaise.

Frozen blueberries and other frozen berries – for desserts and cereal.

STAPLES, STORE LIST
AND KITCHEN EQUIPMENT

Whole-wheat or whole-grain flour and breadcrumbs –
for use in recipes.

Healthy desserts – Low-salt and low-sugar cookies and frozen
non-fat, sugar-free desserts.

Fruit cups – unsweetened applesauce and small containers of
other unsweetened fruits, such as pineapple in cans.

Dried, unsulphured fruits – dates, raisins, apricots, etc.

Unsalted nuts – especially walnuts; also almonds.

Natural peanut butter – with no salt, sugar or other additives.
Walnut and almond butters are also good choices.

Broth – low-sodium, fat-free chicken broth, and vegetable broth
such as Pritikin's.

**Various no-sodium seasoning mixes with no added sugar
or fats** – such as Italian seasoning and Mrs. Dash's, to use in place of
salt in recipes.

Low-fat or fat-free, sugar-free salad dressings – and non-
creamy Italian dressing.

Condiments – sugar-free or low-sugar, low-sodium ketchup; Dijon
mustard rather than regular mustard; low-sodium soy sauce.

Low-sodium, sugar-free or low-sugar tomato products –
tomato paste, tomato sauce, tomato juice and spaghetti sauce.

Some dried herbs and spices – especially those that are difficult
to find fresh.

STAPLES, STORE LIST
AND KITCHEN EQUIPMENT

Preparing a Grocery List

In addition to staples, you will want to purchase fruits and vegetables, breads and juices, so you will need to add them to your grocery list. You will also be buying meat, fish and poultry, as well as some dairy products and other foods.

You want to choose as large a variety of fresh fruits and vegetables as possible for the healthiest possible eating, but not in such large amounts that you risk them spoiling. Bagged salads are a convenient choice and often include a mixture of greens (such as field greens) not usually found loose in an ordinary supermarket. However, loose greens such as romaine and spinach are less expensive and since they are uncut probably retain a higher degree of nutrients. Iceberg lettuce can be used as filler but has very few nutrients.

Vegetables can be kept fresh for some time in your crisper when well wrapped in paper towels. This absorbs moisture from the refrigerator. For foods that do better with moisture, such as mushrooms, wrap or cover them with a damp cloth or damp paper towels. These damp-wrapped items can also be placed in a plastic bag. To refresh vegetables such as celery and carrots that have become limp, place them in a container of iced water in the refrigerator for a few hours.

If fresh vegetables aren't available or practical, then frozen is also a very good choice. Single vegetables such as broccoli or mixed frozen vegetables with no salt or other additives, rather than frozen entrees, are the wisest selections. The majority of frozen dinners and breakfast items, even those that are low in calories, have high sodium and/or sugar content, high saturated fat and other undesirable additives.

There is nothing like the flavor of fresh herbs when you can get them. If you have the inclination, you can grow most of your favorites outside or inside in a window garden, and they don't take much work or space. Many herbs can be purchased fresh at the supermarket, such as garlic, ginger root, basil, oregano, dill and lemon grass. Wrapping paper towels around fresh green herbs will help them stay fresh in the refrigerator. Certain ones, such as chives, can sometimes be found in the supermarket freezer section and are a little more pungent than dried herbs.

Many fresh fruits, such as bananas and peaches, should be purchased just before the ripening stage; otherwise they may spoil before they can be eaten. For best results, purchase only a few days' supply. A few fruits and vegetables will last just about forever, however, such as apples, onions, and sweet potatoes, and often don't even need to be refrigerated if stored in a cool, dry place. Once cut, however, they should be stored in your refrigerator. Fresh citrus juices are wonderful, but pretty good orange juice can be purchased in a carton, and it has often been fortified with calcium and additional vitamin C.

Choose the better cuts of meats and poultry. Lean beef is best, while white meat chicken and turkey, such as the breast portion, is much healthier than dark meat. Be sure to include plenty of fresh or frozen fish, especially fatty fish such as salmon.

What you put on your list is the first step toward getting a healthier diet in place. Your next step is a visit to the grocery store, but make sure you have the right equipment to prepare your healthy meals when you get back. Some suggestions are listed below.

Useful Kitchen Equipment

Knives – It really isn't necessary to have a dozen or so kitchen knives. You can easily get along with just three important ones: a chef's knife to do the chopping and slicing; a paring knife for peeling and detailed cutting; and a serrated knife that will slice through foods such as tomatoes and bread.

You may already have one or more of these knives on hand. But if you don't or you want to buy new ones, you don't have to pay a lot of money for them. Nor do they all have to be a particular brand. You should, however, shop around so you can see which feels the most comfortable for you.

If you can, invest the most money in a chef's knife because it will probably be the utensil you use the most. It has a wide, heavy blade from eight to 14 inches long and the flat side can be used to crush garlic and to transfer ingredients from the cutting board to the pan. The weight of the blade should do the majority of the work but it shouldn't be too heavy or you may get tired when using it over a long period of time. Most cooks use a blade that is eight to 10 inches long, but you should choose the one that seems most like the natural extension of your hand.

You want a paring knife that's two to four inches long, has a sharp point and a flat blade, and is easy to handle. Don't go for a curved blade; that's for decorative carving.

A serrated knife should have a thin, narrow blade – eight to 10 inches is the most useful. Its teeth can actually bite into soft foods so it cuts them better and more easily than most other knives. Don't spend much on a serrated knife because it can't be sharpened and will eventually have to be discarded.

Salad spinner – This will make salad preparation much less of a chore because once the salad ingredients have been washed, they don't have to be dried. Just put them in the spinner with the top on and turn the handle. Presto – the water seeps into the bowl holding the strainer and the vegetables in the strainer are relatively dry and ready to go.

Rice steamer – It doesn't have to be expensive. This tool will take fewer nutrients out of your food and cook more evenly than boiling rice in a pot.

Vegetable steamer – This simple tool is inexpensive and is sold in most grocery stores. Choose one that will fit the pots you have. Steaming instead of boiling helps vegetables retain nutrients.

Food processor – Today it's possible to buy a relatively inexpensive food processor and, considering the time it will save you if you cook a lot, it is well worth the investment. In addition, it will increase the number of ways food can be prepared as well as greatly increase the variety of recipes you can make.

Blender – Most food processors have blender capability, but if you feel you don't want to invest in a food processor, at least get a blender. It will make food preparation easier, not to mention all the tasty and healthy desserts, sauces, salad dressings, fruit smoothies and more you can mix up in it.

Grill pan or electric grill – These can be relatively expensive but are well worth the investment. Choose either a large skillet with parallel ridges deep enough for the fat to drain off or choose one of a number of the popular countertop electric grills. If you choose an electric grill, be sure to open it before purchasing to see whether it is large enough for your needs. The grill skillet has the advantage of being more easily stored and cleaned. The electric grill, however, can be purchased in a variety of sizes and used on your countertop. Many also have a removable front or side section to collect fat run-off. Either works well with just a light spray of cooking oil.

CHAPTER 11

SHOPPING HEALTHY – FINDING THE RIGHT FOODS

In order to eat healthy, it's necessary to buy healthy. The best place to start is by checking out which grocery stores are most appropriate for your needs. Look for those that have a large selection of healthy foods. You should be able to find at least 95 percent of the healthy foods you want in most grocery stores.

Making the right choices isn't as difficult or costly as you might expect. There is no reason the budget for healthy foods should be any higher than the budget for unhealthy foods. In fact, you might find yourself spending less by not purchasing as much of some higher-priced items as you once did, such as steak.

It helps to dress comfortably and have on your walking shoes when shopping. It's also important to have a list prepared to take with you to avoid spur-of-the-moment, sometimes unwise food purchases.

Making healthy food selections is an exercise in comparison shopping. Just as you compare price value on food and other goods, now you're going to learn which are the best values healthwise. To do this, you will put into practice all the lessons you've learned so far, especially about reading labels. It will be time-consuming at first, so allow enough leeway to spend a few minutes scrutinizing what's written on the side of each can or front of each package. With just a little practice, you'll become familiar with most of these products and eventually spend much less time shopping.

Dairy Products

That old standard, American cheese in individual slices, is a simple place to start. It's an important staple in the U.S. diet but, though tasty and high in calcium, it is also usually high in calories, saturated fat and salt. Today, however, many manufacturers have developed cheeses lower in saturated fat in varying degrees, such as reduced-fat, low-fat, part-skim and non-fat. Kraft, for example, has at least three versions of American cheese: regular, 2 percent milk and fat-free. Let's compare them with regard to labels:

1) First, check for the serving size, the total calories in that serving and the percentage of those calories that comes from fat.

2) Then check for the total amount of fat and the breakdown between saturated fat and any other kind of fat. Take notice of what percentage of these fats each serving takes of the FDA's recommended daily allowance (the Daily Value) for a 2,000-calorie diet.

3) Check in the same way for cholesterol, sodium, carbohydrates, vitamins, fiber and minerals such as calcium.

4) Also check the list of ingredients. While this listing doesn't indicate amounts, remember that the ingredients are listed in descending order of how much of it the product contains.

Kraft American Cheese Comparisons Table
Serving Size 1 Slice

Type	Calories	Fat/% DV	Sat. Fat/% DV	Chol./% DV	Sod./% DV	Calc./% DV
Regular	60	4.5 g./7%	2.5 g./13%	15mg./13%	250 mg./10%	20%
2% milk	45	3 g./5%	1.5 g./8%	10mg./3%	260 mg./11%	20%
Fat Free	30	0	0	5mg./1%	250mg./10%	20%

% DV = Percentage of FDA's daily recommendation for a 2,000 calorie diet
Sat. Fat = Saturated fat
Chol. = Cholesterol
Sod. = Sodium
Calc. % DV = the Daily Value only of calcium (no amount listed)
g. = gram
mg. = milligram

A serving size for each package is one slice. If you examine the table shown, there are 60 calories per serving in the regular version, with 40 of those calories coming from fat. There are 4.5 grams of fat, which is

7 percent of the FDA's Daily Value. Of that fat, 2.5 grams are saturated fat, 13 percent of the total daily amount of saturated fat recommended for a 2,000-calorie diet.

The same serving size of Kraft 2 percent milk American cheese has 45 calories, with 25 of them coming from fat. The total fat is 3 grams or 5 percent of the daily value, with 1.5 grams of saturated fat, which brings it down to 8 percent of the Daily Value allowance of saturated fat. Better than regular, but not the best.

The label on Kraft's fat-free American cheese, however, says there is no fat. Without it the calorie count is low, only 30 calories per slice. There's no saturated fat, of course, or any other kind of fat.

You find that the fat-free is lower in cholesterol (5 milligrams or 1 percent of the Daily Value) than the 2-percent-milk American (10 milligrams or 3 percent of the Daily Value), and much less than the regular American (15 milligrams or 13 percent of the Daily Value).

The calcium levels (20 percent), important to know for people who need a high calcium intake, are the same. Most other values, such as carbohydrates, sodium and protein, are the same, or about the same, in all three cheeses. But note that the sodium in all three cheeses, 250 mg., is 10 percent of the daily allowance.

The listing of ingredients is pretty similar for all three cheeses. In the list of ingredients on the fat-free label, however, there is an asterisk beside milkfat, an ingredient not shown on the other two versions. Checking what this indicates, you'll see it says "not a significant source of fat." In other words, there actually is a tiny amount of fat but so little that it doesn't have to be recorded on the Nutrition Facts panel.

If you haven't tried many of these healthier versions of products, such as non-fat cheese, at this stage you probably have some questions. For example, how are these products going to taste compared to the "real" thing. Only you can answer that question, so why not go ahead and try the non-fat or at least the low-fat versions? You'll probably find that some taste fine, others may not be at all palatable to you, and some just take a little getting used to. For example, I have been drinking skim milk for so long that regular milk tastes too rich for me. Once you get used to it, you'll find you can't return to the original product.

By the way, there is a big difference between skim and whole milk, even between skim and 2 percent milk, which becomes obvious by reading the labels. There is a large variety of milk these days in addition to these – for example, there is not only regular chocolate milk, but low-fat chocolate milk, soymilk – which may be beneficial for post-menopausal women – and buttermilk. In packaged form there are even more varieties – for example, rice milk, a good choice for people who are lactose intolerant.

Yogurt is another dairy product where you'll find great variety. There is both a basic food product and a frozen form for dessert. Regular yogurt, found in the dairy case, is usually available in lower-fat or fat-free versions in dozens of flavors, mainly fruits. But a close look at some labels reveals that while these versions taste good enough to fill in for dessert, there's a good reason. Most are fairly high in sugar. Some low-fat yogurts, usually called "light," have artificial sweeteners instead of sugar. There's also just plain non-fat, non-sweetened yogurt, which can be used in a variety of ways.

Frozen yogurts can provide a desirable alternative to ice cream as a dessert, because ice cream is so high in fat, calories and sugar. But calories and sugar are generally still fairly high in many frozen selections of yogurt and should be taken into consideration. However, there are lower fat and sugar combinations available, as well as those sweetened with products other than sugar.

There are also healthier versions of other dairy products, such as low-fat and non-fat cottage cheese and ricotta, and other cheeses, even a part-skim mozzarella, which indicates on the package that it now melts more easily than it used to. This should make it easier to use for cooking and making sauces.

Some other healthier versions of dairy products are also great for cooking, or can be used to easily make healthy substitutes, such as non-fat yogurt cheese instead of cream cheese or butter as a spread. You can also make it yourself, as we explain later in this section on nutrition.

There's nothing out there that can truly compare to real butter. Unfortunately, it's often totally solid, meaning totally saturated fat – and often salted. Whipped butter is a better choice. Margarine, once touted as the answer to the butter problem, is no better – it's full of trans fat, and besides, it can't touch butter in the taste category. There are, however, several butter substitutes that are far healthier and tastier choices than margarine and have been gaining acceptance in the past several years.

Eggs are actually healthy foods in many ways, but high in cholesterol, important to know for people who have a cholesterol problem. Egg replacement products, such as EggBeaters™, are available, as well as some made of egg whites only. Eliminating the yolk means eliminating the cholesterol.

Juice, Sports Drinks and Other Beverages

Juices can contribute to the servings of fruit and vegetables that it's important to have each day. However, juices usually have no fiber, while whole fruits and vegetables have a significant amount. And while few canned or frozen citrus juices can measure up to the taste of freshly squeezed orange and grapefruit juices, many kinds are nutritionally OK – if they are made totally from juice. But it's important to check for added sugar and/or sodium content.

Here are three interesting juices you might want to add to your diet: unsweetened Concord grape juice, blueberry juice and pomegranate juice, including combinations such as pomegranate mango and cherry, all full of antioxidants and flavonoids.

Frozen juice concentrates and orange or grapefruit juices in cartons compare favorably for nutrition with fresh juices. Several also have added calcium and other vitamins, which make them pretty healthy choices. Some even include pulp, the most nutritious part of the orange.

Few regular supermarkets carry fresh-squeezed juices. The best place to find these are usually fruit or produce stands or fresh markets. Fresh-squeezed orange juice also often includes some healthy pulp. However, most freshly squeezed juices are not put through the pasteurization process, which sterilizes them.

Vegetable juices are difficult to find other than in a bottle or can, except perhaps at a juice bar, where you may find fresh carrot juice and other vegetable juices, sometimes blended together. Good choices in canned vegetable juices are low-sodium tomato juices and low-sodium V-8, which contains a variety of vegetables and can be used to make sauces.

Sports drinks may be popular but they are high in sugar with little nutritional value. They're basically designed for people doing very long or strenuous exercise sessions. Plain water or bottled water is a much better choice.

For the most part, stay away from sodas (soft drinks), with the exception of club soda. Like sports drinks, sodas have little food value but may have lots of sugar. They also may have caffeine. One of the biggest problems with these drinks is that many people tend to consume them to the exclusion of other, healthier beverages. So if you must have one, then just have one occasionally and try to drink sugar-free or at least caffeine-free or both, and still drink plenty of water and healthy juices. Or try drinking green or black tea, which both have many benefits. The caffeine content in teas and soft drinks is lower than that of coffee.

Condiments

Like many food products, condiments frequently have a high sodium content and may have quite a bit of sugar as well. Fortunately, there are low-sodium versions of both soy sauce and ketchup. And while regular mustard has sodium, Dijon mustard contains none. If you buy honey Dijon mustard, however, the honey in it does contain sugar.

Vegetables

Are canned vegetables up to par with fresh or even frozen? Canned no-sodium or low-sodium tomatoes, whole or diced, and tomato sauces are just about as good as fresh tomatoes. They're actually better in some ways because they've been cooked, which releases the lycopene, an important antioxidant in tomatoes. But beware of high sugar content in some.

It's best to scrutinize most canned vegetables carefully because of possible high sodium content, saturated fats and added sugars. This also can be true of soups, by the way. Nowadays, there are several healthier versions available, including the Pritikin line.

Almost every vegetable that can be found in the produce section can also be found frozen, including green beans, spinach, broccoli, asparagus and mixed vegetables, a good choice for stir-fry dishes and homemade soups. They are usually frozen right after harvest, so they may actually be as fresh or even fresher than vegetable produce you buy at the market.

Where people often run into problems with frozen vegetables is when there are more than just vegetables in the package. Some contain additives, creamy sauces and lots of fat, sodium and/or sugar.

When it comes to fresh vegetables, color is the key – bright red, green, yellow and even orange peppers, green-as-grass broccoli, dark leafy spinach and mustard greens, the darker lettuces, bright purple radicchio and deep red cabbage. You'll want to examine these carefully to make sure they're fresh.

Some vegetables, such as green beans, often come in packages that may be more than you need. Since vegetables should always be as fresh as possible, ask a store employee to open a bag or package for you so you can take a smaller portion more suited to your needs. For convenience, you might also want to try a bag of varied salad greens, which are often pre-washed.

It's best to steer clear of white vegetables, except for garlic, cauliflower and onions. But since potatoes are one of the top foods in the American diet, let's look at the ways to fix them that are the healthiest. If you must eat potatoes, I suggest baked, grilled or broiled – not fried. Eat the nutritious skin and avoid all but the lowest-fat condiments. Later in the book, you'll find out how to make healthy potato wedges, which have little actual potato except the skin and make a great substitute for hash browns or french fries.

Fruits

When you're shopping, take a look at fresh fruits and try to determine their freshness and how close they are to being ripe. Again, you are looking for texture, color and firmness. The "no-white" rule also applies here – no coconuts, for example, because they are high in unhealthy oil.

Today produce comes from all over the world, including the Southern Hemisphere. Much of it is available during the winter season in the Northern Hemisphere. Other produce comes from tropical climates and is available year-round.

Frozen fruits can be great alternatives to fresh fruit, especially frozen berries, among the healthiest of foods. Like fresh and frozen vegetables, they are often in better shape when frozen than fresh berries sometimes are by the time they arrive at the supermarket. You can find a good variety – strawberries, raspberries, blackberries and, of course, blueberries – one of the "10 best foods."

Now we come to canned fruits, a place where people run into trouble because the majority of canned fruits have added sugar, lots of it. Examine the labels and you'll see several examples of this, including canned peaches in thick syrup and canned mandarin oranges. There are some good choices of unsweetened canned fruit, however, such as pineapple.

Snacks

Normally I would suggest that when you're shopping, you should completely skip the snack sections – as in potato chips, candy, cookies and crackers. If you don't go that route, you won't be tempted. But it's important to learn how they compare with healthy snacks. When you do, you'll be amazed at some of the differences.

Crackers are a good example. Although it usually takes quite a few to build up a lot of calories, most aren't really healthy foods, due to high sodium, saturated-fat and trans-fat content. Only a few labels now list the amount of trans fat, so it's important to check the list of ingredients in various crackers, candies, desserts and other foods. Chances are that most show partially hydrogenated vegetable oils as an ingredient. Low-fat cookies may still have high sugar and sodium, and some brands have triggered allergies in some people.

Many snacks that are considered healthy, even touted as such by the manufacturers, may not be healthy in some ways. Popcorn is a good example. Air popped, without butter, it's about as healthy a snack as can be found. But add butter, salt and maybe a little sugar, and it's a different story. Most microwave brands also have trans fat.

But there are lots of truly healthy snacks available. Canned or packaged unsweetened applesauce, especially berry and applesauce combinations – which have lots of phytochemicals and come in individual serving sizes – make great snacks.

Broccoli florets, baby carrots, celery sticks, apples and other raw fruits and veggies also make good snacks. I store them in small plastic bags in my refrigerator so I can grab a packet to take with me on my way out the door.

Cereals

There is an overwhelming amount of mixtures, types and brands of cereals available. Oatmeal – yes, the old-fashioned, takes-time-to-cook kind, not the instant – is one of the best choices. I recommend McCann's Irish oatmeal, which is tasty, filling and satisfying. I like mine with both white and dark raisins and a little skim milk. Adding walnuts is another option. I usually have a week's supply made up and stored in the refrigerator; then I can just microwave as much as I want for breakfast.

Shredded Wheat, Cheerios and Grape-Nuts are all good choices, as well. But many cereals, although enriched, still don't have all the essential nutrients lost in refining and are heavy on added sugar. These are not the ones you want to have for breakfast or a snack.

Rice

Pastas, bread and rice are grains as well. But white rice, which is refined, and instant rice products, which also have been processed, are not healthy choices. Better are unrefined, unbleached brown rice, wild rice or mixtures such as brown and wild rice, which are made up of complex carbohydrates and still retain their fiber. An especially tasty and healthy choice is brown basmati rice, full of flavor. When cooked, it tastes naturally almost like butter has been added.

Pasta

There are dozens of different pastas – linguini, egg noodles, elbow macaroni, fettuccini, multicolored spinach or tomato pasta. Try to avoid refined white pastas. Instead, look for whole-grain pasta products, such as whole wheat – stone ground if you can find it.

There are several choices of blended pastas, such as Ronzoni's Healthy Harvest whole-wheat blend rotini, which contains whole-wheat flour and some semolina, made from refined, enriched white flour of protein-rich durham wheat. These are good transitional choices for people adding fiber to their diet.

Breads

Bread – the staff of life. Without it, where would we be? But I'm sure what the philosopher had in mind was not the bread of the 20th century – white, refined and not very nutritious, even the enriched and low-calorie loaves we see today. Like other grains, bread is best when unrefined and made of whole grain, and there are several choices in addition to whole wheat. If it is stone ground and/or reduced calorie, all the better. Whole-wheat pita, without transfatty acids, is also a good choice.

Nuts

Nuts are a very healthy food, as long as they are not salted. They are great sources of omega-3 fatty acids, especially walnuts. They not only make a good snack but also can be used to add interest to many foods, such as salads and desserts. However, it's important to eat nuts in small portions, as they are also high in calories – some much more than others. While peanuts are actually legumes, they have been included in this section, since they offer many of the same benefits as nuts.

A word about peanut butter: All versions are high in fat, especially saturated fat, and some have added sugar. Also, even reduced-fat versions are another source of hidden trans fat. Sure enough, when you check the labels, you'll see that partially hydrogenated oils are included in the list of ingredients. If you want to have peanut butter, better choices are "natural" peanut butters, which also contain saturated fat but consist of only peanuts, although some brands have a little salt. They do taste different than what you may be used to – they actually taste like peanuts! Consider giving them a try. Since they contain no additives to bind the oil and thick nut base, they do have to be stirred before you eat them. They may have to be purchased at a health food store or fresh market if your grocery store doesn't carry them.

Legumes

Legumes – peas, beans, lentils and peanuts – are pretty healthy foods. Most, except peanuts, are low in calories, are high in incomplete protein and dietary fiber and other nutrients, and are also filling. They can be canned, dried and even frozen and can be used in a variety of ways.

Salad Dressings

If you can't eat a salad without dressing, there are dozens of low-fat and non-fat dressing options available today. While most fat-free Italian dressings are sugar-free, many other low-fat dressings do have added sugars, which can be a surprisingly high amount. You'll also need to watch out for sodium content in some. You may want to make your own salad dressings. You'll find recipes for some quick and easy ones in this book.

SHOPPING HEALTHY –
FINDING THE RIGHT FOODS

Cooking Sprays

All liquid oils do have some saturated fat, but some have less and are also high in polyunsaturated and monounsaturated fats, considered much healthier. You need some of these fats in your diet. To cut down on the overall amount of oils in your diet, however, consider using cooking sprays. Flavored sprays are fine, too, also very low in calories and fat, and can add interest to foods cooked with them. Never, never, never use any form of solid – that means saturated fat and trans fat – shortening. And although you may have been brought up using it, do away completely with chicken fat, bacon fat, and, of course, lard in your diet!

Seafood

Fresh fish must be just that – fresh. If it smells the least bit fishy, walk away. If it doesn't, look for other indications of whether fish and other seafood are fresh.

While fresh fish and shellfish may be the ultimate seafood experience, frozen fish can be very good. But the only way you can know for certain is to just take a chance and try them.

But you want to be careful about processed frozen seafood, which is often breaded. Also, checking the labels of frozen dinners with seafood, you can see that the overall content, which may include several additives, sauces, white rice, macaroni and cheese, etc., makes them not such good choices.

Canned fish, especially tuna and salmon, have been staples in a variety of dishes for years. Solid white tuna packed in water is a good choice. And don't forget sardines and herring, high in omega-3s – but watch out for the amount of sodium. I like Rubenstein's fancy blueback red salmon from a can, which has multiple uses: as an addition to salads, in salmon croquettes and in salmon mousse, used as a dip. Both tuna and salmon now come in a foil packet, which many people seem to prefer.

Beef and Other Red Meats

Many of today's meats are much leaner than they were even 20 years ago. Although some people lament what they say these products have lost in flavor, the benefits may be worth it, since lower saturated fats in the diet can help prevent heart disease, diabetes and other serious diseases. So stay with the healthiest cuts of meat. It's also good to strictly limit red meat in your diet, but if you're in the mood for beef more than once in a while, always choose the leanest cuts. And don't hesitate to ask the butcher to trim the fat.

I stay away from almost all red meat, except when I indulge myself two or three times a year and have the best steak I can find! But I always ask to have the fat removed and the gravy drained off.

Ah, hamburgers and hot dogs, those great all-American foods. Some cuts of ground beef have less fat than others, but try ground turkey – it should be from white meat – which can be lower in fat than regular hamburger, even ground sirloin. You might find you like it just as well or better than ground beef. Also, why not try ground soy meat, and some soy and vegetable combinations?

What can be said about hot dogs? You know they aren't good for you but sometimes you just have to have one. So pick the healthiest kind you can find, such as fat-free Oscar Meyer or turkey hot dogs. It's hard to find them without high salt content, however, which is of concern for people with high blood pressure or on a low-salt diet for other reasons.

Poultry

When buying poultry, skinless breasts are the best choice, as white meat is far healthier and has less fat than dark meat, and the skin has too much saturated fat. To reduce the cost, you can also choose regular chicken breasts, with skins and bone in, and remove the skin yourself. You will need to carefully examine the package to make sure the chicken is of good color and firm. Frozen boneless chicken breasts are also usually readily available.

Canned poultry is convenient and requires no cooking. This can be a good choice, especially for sandwiches and salads. There are a few brands of canned chicken on the market, but you see more chicken combinations, such as chicken and dumplings. Look at these labels for sodium, saturated fat and cholesterol. You may be surprised to find out just how high those contents are.

Most chicken in the regular frozen food section seems to be part of a frozen chicken entree or chicken-based dish. Again, look at these labels and you'll find high sodium, fat and cholesterol counts in many of them.

By now you should have a pretty good idea of what to look for to purchase healthy foods, and there are a number of healthy recipes in the back of the book to help you create healthy and tasty meals.

SHOPPING HEALTHY –
FINDING THE RIGHT FOODS

Dos and Don'ts for Shopping for Healthy Foods

- Do select grocery stores carefully based on the availability of healthy foods, the freshest produce and knowledgeable attendants.

- Don't walk into the supermarket without making a detailed list of the specific items you need before you go shopping; otherwise, you'll pick up extraneous, often unhealthy items.

- Do allow yourself enough time to spend on shopping, which includes reading labels. Wear comfortable clothes and shoes, and be sure to eat before going so you're not shopping while you're hungry and more likely to make bad choices.

- Do read ingredient listings and nutritional labels, and remember that ingredients are listed in order of their quantity in the food.

- Don't use any products that contain hydrogenated or partially hydrogenated vegetable oils.

- Do choose bright colors and firm textures in fresh fruits and vegetables.

- Don't go to the aisles stocked with candy, soda, chips, etc.

- Do choose healthy convenience items, such as cut fresh fruit and vegetables, bagged salad greens and healthy snack foods.

- Do choose the leanest cuts of meat and poultry. Acquaint yourself with the butcher so he or she can accommodate your needs on each visit.

- Do carefully select seafood. Fresh is better than frozen and deep-sea fish are better than farmed.

CHAPTER 12

PREPARING HEALTHY SNACKS

Three a Day

Having healthy snacks on hand is a good way to avoid the hunger that can lead to overeating or snacking on unhealthy foods, especially if you eat relatively small portions at meals as I do.

There's a problem, however, with buying snacks other than fruits and vegetables at the supermarket because so few pre-packaged ones are healthy choices. Most of them, in fact, are very unhealthy. For example, most microwave popcorn and crackers contain trans fat in the form of partially hydrogenated oils or vegetable shortening.

Yet there is such a wide variety of healthy snack food available, usually so simple and easy to prepare and tasting so good, that it isn't necessary to resort to unhealthy snacks from the grocery store.

I usually have three snacks a day – at mid-morning, mid-afternoon and a couple of hours after dinner. When I'm at home I often like to eat a slice or two of whole-grain, raisin-walnut toast with non-fat yogurt cheese between breakfast and lunch. It's tasty, filling and nutritious and keeps me satisfied until it's time for the next meal. At other times, I vary my morning snack by having fruit – for example, a half cup of watermelon.

My afternoon snack often consists of an apple or other fruit. Frequently, I have a combination of foods, such as a half cup of melon and three fat-free Fig Newtons, which I like very much.

I don't skimp on desserts as snacks, especially in the evening, but I choose non-fat items generally sweetened with Splenda. I especially enjoy fat-free, sugar-free frozen fudge bars. They taste great and don't have anything in them that I should avoid.

Take Them Along

One snack I often have is a healthy trail mix made up at the house and stored in pre-measured amounts in plastic bags. Ingredients vary but usually include foods such as seeds, dry unrefined cereals, and a handful of nuts and perhaps just a little dried fruit – since both nuts and dried fruit are high in calories. All of these products are good for me. Nuts provide omega-3 fatty acids, fruits provide antioxidants, cereal provides fiber, and seeds provide various other nutrients.

As you can see, I usually prefer fruit over vegetables for snacks, but people who love foods from the vegetable garden have a lot of very good selections to choose from. Raw broccoli, celery, carrots and cauliflower can be cut up and packaged in plastic bags in advance.

The advantage to many of these snacks, whether it's trail mix, vegetables or certain fruits such as grapes and bananas, is that with very little preparation they can be taken with you just about anywhere you go. I often stuff an apple or other snack in my pocket on my way out the door. I can eat it after exercising, on a walk, in the car or elsewhere when I get the urge. That's why the smell of hot dogs at the ballpark doesn't bother me a bit. It's great to be able to munch on a bag of trail mix at the game instead of giving in to the urge to eat french fries or pizza.

A Variety of Other Good Snack Choices

Another good snack almost any time of day at home is a bowl of cereal with skim milk and half a banana or a tablespoon of raisins. A cup of unsweetened canned applesauce or crushed pineapple is also a healthy option. Mix the pineapple with a little non-fat cottage cheese or try mixing vegetables into it such as diced peppers, cherry tomatoes and scallions.

Non-fat "yogurt cheese," either purchased at the grocery store or made at home by straining plain, non-fat yogurt through a mesh strainer and letting it sit in the refrigerator overnight, can be used to stuff celery or spread over Melba toast. A small amount of natural peanut butter can also be used as a stuffing or spread. The yogurt cheese can be used as a dip for carrots or other raw veggies. To drink, choose black, or even better, green iced tea with a bit of lemon or lime. Up to eight ounces of fresh or canned unsweetened, low-sodium fruit and vegetable juices are also good choices.

Baked sweet potatoes, sliced in the shape of french fries and moistened with a little olive oil and a dash of sun salt, and broiled until crisp, make a great at-home snack. So do roasted potato wedges, cooked in a similar way (see recipe section). Both are a healthy substitute for french fries.

Plain sugar-free, non-fat yogurt is a great base for a healthy snack. Just add blueberries, strawberries or other berries to a cup of it and mix it together. Or use a combination of berries and cut-up fruit such as peaches. Non-fat yogurt with a little artificial sweetener also makes a great topping for fruits and other healthy snacks – much better for you than whipped cream!

A slice of homemade cake or pie made without sugar and saturated fat can make a great dessert snack. For example, it's possible to make a spice cake by substituting unsweetened applesauce in place of vegetable shortening or unhealthy oils. The cake still turns out tasty and moist, as long as you follow the other directions on the recipe.

If you have to wash down your (non-fat, sugar-free) cookies with milk, or dunk them like you did when you were a kid, do yourself a favor and try them with skim milk, soymilk or even rice milk. These are much healthier than whole milk and aren't going to add bad fats to your diet. You also might want to try dunking them in a cup of hot green or black tea instead.

How about a half sandwich on whole-wheat bread with non-fat cheddar cheese and Dijon mustard? To make it more interesting, try layering it with slices of peppers, onion and fresh spinach.

Here's another great idea for a healthy snack in lieu of potato chips. It only takes about 10 minutes to make and isn't labor-intensive. Cut a slice of whole-wheat pita bread into triangles and brush them with garlic powder, a little Italian seasoning and a little olive oil. Bake them in the oven for about five minutes and you have a tray of hot, crunchy treats. These also have the advantage of other snacks on the go because they can be stored in plastic bags once they've cooled.

You can see that an endless variety of foods can be used for healthy snacks. As long as the foods are ones that are good for you and the portions are moderate, it only takes your imagination to come up with ones that will stave off hunger and help keep you healthy at the same time.

CHAPTER 13

NUTRITION AWAY FROM HOME

When you're at home, you're able to control what you eat. You can shop for healthy alternatives and avoid temptation by not buying foods that are harmful to your health. But what about when you're away from home? If you have choices – healthy or unhealthy – the decisions you make are critical. You have more choices, however, than you might realize.

Restaurants

When you're at a restaurant, you can usually find something healthy on the menu that you will enjoy. Sometimes, however, foods that are otherwise healthy aren't prepared in the healthiest way. Grilled chicken and seafood, for example, may not be as healthy as you think in a restaurant because they may have a coating of butter or an oil/butter combination to keep them from sticking to the grill. Don't be shy. Ask your server how it is cooked, and if it's not coated with a healthy oil, such as olive oil, ask if you can have it prepared that way or if you can get it dry. Otherwise, you may be getting an unexpected dose of saturated fat and/or trans fat.

If the fish comes with a lemon-butter sauce, you can ask for lemon only instead. There are other changes you can request, such as asking that vegetables be served unbuttered and/or steamed. Forego the french fries and have double or triple orders of vegetables or salads instead. Offer to pay for it if you wish, but chances are you won't be charged extra.

Ask for non-fat, low-sugar salad dressings or simply oil and vinegar – and be sure to ask for it on the side. Another idea is to ask for a mixture of Dijon mustard and balsamic vinegar and make up your own dressing.

Sauces too, especially creamy ones, can make a big difference in how much saturated fat or trans fat you take in. Avoid them when you can or eat only a small amount.

Fill up on the healthier elements of a meal, such as the salad, and don't feel you have to clean your plate. Take home what's left if you really want it and skip dessert or ask for fresh fruit instead.

If you are planning to dine in a restaurant that requires reservations, you may want to make your requests known when you make the reservations. I've found many restaurants are happy to accommodate special needs if they know in advance. If they can't accommodate your needs when you ask in advance, pick another restaurant.

What if you go to a restaurant and find there's nothing on the menu you like that fits into a healthy eating lifestyle? I would say, first of all, to avoid these restaurants whenever possible; your friends will probably understand and be amenable if you tell them your reasons. However, if you're faced with this situation unexpectedly, there are a few things you can do. Order the least-unhealthy item you see and eat only enough to keep from being hungry. While it isn't possible in some eateries, ask if there is anything that can be made, such as a large salad, that can be substituted for what's on the menu. You may be surprised to learn it's something that can be done and that the restaurant is only too happy to do it for you.

I'd like to add that, while fast-food restaurants have been adding healthier foods to their menus, most still are not very healthy and it can be difficult to find out just how much fat, sugar or sodium is contained in the foods there.

The Breakfast Buffet – A Danger Zone

While any buffet menu can provide temptation to eat unhealthy foods, the breakfast buffet deserves special attention, whether you're just going out for breakfast in your hometown, or staying in a hotel, motel or elsewhere. Breakfast buffets are often part of the room package these days, so you may feel obligated to eat from them in the hotel dining room. And there they are, all those fattening, sweet, loaded-with-saturated-fat foods that you seldom have at home.

The best way to deal with a breakfast buffet is to go right past the meats, cheeses and pastries and try not to look. Head for the fruits, which are usually fresh, and load up your plate. Add a bowl of oatmeal or cold cereal and use non-fat milk if it's available. If you want bread, pass up the corn muffins for whole-wheat toast and take only a packet of jelly. If you decide you want eggs, and there is an omelet chef, ask for one made with egg whites or EggBeaters™. There are usually lots of interesting items that can be added, such as peppers and onions.

Then – don't go back for a refill.

Eating at Someone Else's Home

This is somewhat trickier because the last thing you want to do is to offend any of your friends or family members. But it's my feeling that they'd much rather prepare something you can eat and enjoy before you arrive than to learn when you get there that the meal they planned is not the kind of food you wish to eat. Once you're there, it will be much more difficult, not to mention inconvenient for your hosts, to prepare a special dish for you.

So call ahead and explain your situation, telling them there's no need to prepare a special dish just for you, that something like a simple salad or vegetables will do.

You may want to be more flexible if you're invited to a holiday meal because it is usually a traditional one with certain meats, vegetables and desserts that are special to the host. In this case, there is frequently a wide choice of foods and you will generally find some that are healthier than others. But since it's a special occasion, you don't have to forego eating the candied yams or the stuffing, for example, but take less of them and more of the healthier foods. In addition, you can sometimes lessen the damage. For example, remove the skin from the turkey and go easy on the gravy. Have dessert but take a small portion.

How to Eat Healthy While Traveling

By Car

It's not hard to maintain a healthy diet when traveling in the car, because you have the opportunity to plan your meals ahead of time and take them with you. You will want to take mainly foods that don't spoil easily, including those that don't need to be kept cold and/or those that can be stored in a cooler for a day or so. Spoilable items can usually be purchased along the way and eaten soon afterward.

Prepare salads and similar foods ahead of time and, for convenience, you may want to store them in disposable containers. Don't take along foods that have to be mixed together on the road because that may prove difficult if there's no place to do it. Be sure to make up some healthy snacks in advance and bring along durable fruits such as apples and pears. This way, when you have to stop for ice or gas, you won't be so hungry that you end up with a package or two of Twinkies from the convenience store.

Also, take along plenty of water, a few gallons at least. Use the ice from your cooler or store ice from your refrigerator in a plastic bag in the cooler. Take along some juices and make up a batch of green or iced tea.

If you travel a lot by car or go great distances, you may want to invest in a small portable refrigerator that can be charged by a car cigarette lighter while traveling. These aren't too expensive and can be taken from the car when you reach your accommodations or stop for the night and plugged into an ordinary electrical outlet.

Eating your own meals on the road can be an enjoyable experience, especially if the weather is warm enough to eat outdoors at a roadside picnic area, where you can get some exercise and enjoy nature as well.

By Plane

Unless you're traveling by private jet or going first class, most flights within the continental United States no longer offer meals that are included in the cost of airfare. Yes, you get a drink and a snack, which usually consists of cookies, pretzels or cheese and a couple of crackers – all no-no's because of trans fat, salt and sugar. It's easy enough to bring your own healthy foods. For a short trip, you may want to bring only snacks that won't spoil. These can be carried in a purse or even a briefcase and are available whenever hunger strikes.

On longer trips, bring more, but prepare these in advance. A whole-grain sandwich of turkey and greens with mustard will probably remain fresh long enough for you to have it as a meal. This is especially important when you have a layover. While major airports usually have a wide selection of restaurants, they may not include eateries with healthy foods. In addition, if your layover is short and/or food lines are long, you may not have time to find something healthy to eat, even if you plan to take it with you on the next leg of your flight. Also, if you have your own food, you can always eat it in-flight.

While a few airlines have started serving food and charging for it, your best bet still may be to take your own, not only for your health but for your taste buds. It may be possible to find out in advance what food is available for a particular flight, but that information won't tell you how good it's going to taste or what's in it.

If you do get meals on your flight, talk to your reservation agent or have your travel agent call ahead and request that a healthy meal be set aside for you. The airlines have many requests for special meals, and it's routine for them to make these arrangements.

By Train or Bus

Trains geared for fairly lengthy travel usually have meals available in the dining car. However, meals are generally served within a relatively short time frame and not always when you want to eat. So some carry-on snacks that won't spoil may be in order.

Shorter train trips don't usually feature a dining car, so it's important to take enough snacks and food to keep you from being hungry on the trip. Some trains may have snack machines but you can't be sure there will be any food available that's healthy. Don't forget to bring something to drink. If you don't mind carrying one, take along a small cooler to keep beverages cold. Another option is to bring a thermos bottle containing water or hot or cold beverages.

Eating healthy snacks to keep from being hungry while traveling can be difficult on a bus tour because most meals are prearranged at scheduled stops. During free periods you generally have a selection of places to dine. But you still may want to take with you some healthy snacks that won't spoil.

Talk to your travel agent or tour operator to learn whether it's possible to arrange for healthy meals of your choice in advance. If it's not, or you don't wish to do this, just follow the guidelines for healthy eating in restaurants and you won't go back home weighing more than you did when you began your trip.

By Ship

Ah, cruises – those hotbeds of temptation. This is probably where it is easiest to forget about eating healthy and go overboard by overeating, especially all the wrong things. There are usually at least six meals a day, counting mid-morning snacks, afternoon tea and a midnight buffet in addition to regular meals. The problem is that, for many people, eating is half the fun of being on a cruise.

There are some things you can do without giving up a lot of the pleasure. First of all, talk to your travel agent about the kinds of meals you want to eat. It's usually possible to arrange healthy meals in advance.

Once aboard, do as you would do in any restaurant and be part of the "Don't Clean Your Plate Club."

Find out in advance about programs on board that involve exercise, the kind you think you can do. Excellent gyms with good equipment are frequently available and exercise programs such as aerobics are often offered. You can also dance, play shuffleboard, swim in the pool and take walks around the deck several times a day. Sign up for excursions on shore where you can walk. Go snorkeling if you're up to it. Exercise will help balance out any overindulgences, and it can take you away from the temptations of those extra meals.

This is definitely the time to try my suggestion about eating just a few bites of those enticing desserts and leaving most of them in the bowl or on the plate.

CHAPTER 14

NUTRITION CONCERNS
FOR SENIORS

What are some of the most significant nutritional concerns for seniors that may not apply to the general population? What unhealthy conditions are exacerbated by poor nutrition, and how can good nutrition aid seniors to avoid some of these conditions? Let's take a look.

According to many studies, a surprising number of seniors suffer from malnutrition, either from eating too many unhealthy foods or from not eating enough healthy foods, or both, or from simply not eating enough. These can all contribute to numerous health problems for which seniors are particularly at risk.

Osteoporosis

As people get older, they tend to lose bone mass. While exercise is a major way to slow down this process, nutrition also plays an important part. The loss of bone mass can eventually lead to osteoporosis, a condition in which bones that have become fragile and porous can break easily. Broken bones are a major risk factor for seniors and, in fact, can lead not only to disability but, in the case of broken hips, also frequently to death in older people. Although post-menopausal women are most at risk, many men have osteoporosis as well.

As most of us know, calcium is a major factor in building and maintaining strong bones. How can we attain the calcium we need from food and still eat healthy? There are several good options.

One of the best ways is to stick to non-fat or at least low-fat dairy products. Skim milk on cereal or non-fat mozzarella in a casserole doesn't make much difference in taste. And there are other healthy dairy sources of calcium available. One very good choice is non-fat, sugar-free yogurt, which generally supplies from 20 percent to 30 percent of the recommended daily amount of calcium for those eating about 2,000 calories a day. It can be purchased with fruit and sweetener for a dessert-like treat, or purchased plain and then sweetened at home by adding fresh or unsweetened canned fruit. A little artificial sweetener can also be added.

Today, many products have been fortified with calcium, including cereals and canned and packaged orange juice. Other products containing added calcium can be substituted for dairy products, such as soy or rice milk, which come in a variety of flavors. Keep an eye out for sugar content, however.

Many vegetables, such as broccoli, spinach, Brussels sprouts and cabbage, can help supply needed calcium. Beans and whole grains, dried figs and apples, and Brazil nuts and almonds are good sources as well.

Calcium also has other jobs to do related to good health, such as helping muscles work. One problem for seniors, however, is that they sometimes have trouble absorbing calcium. Others, particularly post-menopausal women, may not get enough calcium (a minimum of 1,200 mg. daily is the recommended amount) from food, and people with osteoporosis and those with low bone mass need even more calcium, even if they are taking osteoporosis medication. These people can get additional needed calcium from mineral supplements.

To work well, calcium needs vitamin D. The best way to get it is through sunlight. It only takes about 15 to 20 minutes of sunshine two or three days a week to supply the necessary amount, but sunscreen will block it out. Sitting inside with sunlight shining through the window doesn't help, because the glass prevents vitamin D from forming. It can be a particular problem when bad winter weather makes it difficult for seniors to get out, especially for those who fear falling when walking on ice or on snow-covered streets.

There are some good food sources of vitamin D, however, such as papaya and red raspberries. See the Vitamin and Minerals chapter for more choices. Vitamin D is also sometimes added to calcium supplements to help the calcium do its work.

Vitamin C, magnesium, manganese and phosphorus also are important in promoting healthy bones and teeth. Vitamin C is found mainly in fruits and vegetables. Magnesium helps assimilate vitamin C and calcium and can be found in many foods including whole grains, legumes, fruits, vegetables and nuts. Like vitamin D, it is often added to calcium supplements.

Manganese helps to strengthen bones and is found in green leafy vegetables, citrus fruits, whole grains and the skin of nuts. Phosphorous, which helps to promote growth of bones and teeth, is found in dozens of foods: whole grains of all kinds, various nuts and seeds, beans, fruits and vegetables like garlic, yams and mushrooms.

As you can see, the foods mentioned that help ward off osteoporosis are part of a healthy diet and are beneficial in warding off other diseases as well.

Heart Disease

Although young adults and even children are susceptible to heart disease, it is mainly a disease of older people, often materializing as early as in their 50s. While many women are most concerned about breast cancer, once they pass menopause their rate of death from heart disease as they age begins to climb until it is on the same level as that of men. It is the leading cause of death for older members of both genders in America and most Western countries.

So it is just as important for senior women to guard against heart disease by maintaining healthy nutrition as it is for senior men. Both genders need to make sure they are getting enough antioxidants, avoiding unhealthy fats, getting a good share of healthy fats, and getting plenty of the B vitamins, many of which play a major role in good heart health. Check the Vitamin and Mineral chapter for additional information.

Pernicious Anemia

When we think of anemia, we usually think of an iron deficiency. But that is only one kind of anemia. Iron helps to form hemoglobin, which carries oxygen from the lungs to body cells. Anemia is a condition in which blood is deficient in quantity, in hemoglobin or in red blood cells. Seniors, of course, can become anemic from an iron deficiency but we are far more susceptible to pernicious anemia, a lack of enough red blood cells. It can leave us pale and weak and in extreme cases cause irregular heartbeat, a risky condition.

Folic acid and vitamins B6 and B12 all help to form red blood cells. But people can acquire pernicious anemia as they age because vitamin B12 often becomes hard to digest and use.

Other causes of B12 deficiency can lead to pernicious anemia. One is very high consumption of caffeine, which can deplete the body of vitamin B12. In some instances, seniors do not get enough meat, the major source of B12, or they may be vegans, who eat no meat. While there are a few vegetables that have been cited as sources of vitamin B12, scientific research has not discovered a way to access it. When people can no longer digest vitamin B12, B12 supplements can help. One method used to control pernicious anemia is periodic injections of vitamin B12. In addition, some physicians prescribe high doses of B12, often packaged together with vitamin B6 and folic acid in pill form.

Osteoarthritis

The term arthritis actually refers to a group of more than 100 rheumatic diseases and conditions that can cause pain, stiffness and swelling in the joints.

We have all heard of, or perhaps know someone who has, rheumatoid arthritis, a chronic and frequently severe autoimmune disease that can strike anyone at any age, even young children. It is a condition in which the cartilage and tissue in and around the joints has been either damaged or destroyed, and it can have many serious effects, such as anemia, weight loss, fever, and extreme and crippling pain.

On the other hand, the risk of getting osteoarthritis, the other major kind of arthritis, usually increases with age, joint trauma, obesity and repetitive joint use. It's a disease, especially of the weight-bearing joints, that develops when the joint linings degenerate, and can lead to bone spurs, pain and decreased mobility and functioning. Cartilage degeneration is the main feature. Deficient cartilage repair, joint-bone problems and, later in life, inflammation can all contribute to this degeneration and erosion, but sometimes the cause is unknown.

According to the Arthritis Foundation, while those under the age of 45 don't often get osteoarthritis, about 21 million people in this country have it. It has the highest incidence of all diseases, with almost everyone over 60 having some degree of it. Certainly not all cases are severe, and some people have such mild symptoms they're hardly aware of them. But for other people, their osteoarthritis is so bad that the slightest movement is agonizing. Five million Americans per year are disabled by osteoarthritis, the primary cause of lost time from work, and it is responsible for about 7 million doctor visits annually, to the tune of an estimated $86 million loss to the U.S. economy.

Because osteoarthritis is primarily a concern of aging, some nutritional advice that is believed to help with this kind of arthritis is included in this chapter. And, as obesity is also a contributing factor because it puts additional pressure on the joints, it's important we all try to maintain a healthy weight in order to help prevent the onset of osteoarthritis or slow it down.

A 2004 study called the ADAPT trial at Wake Forest University in North Carolina put subjects with osteoarthritis of the knee on a restricted diet coupled with moderate exercise. The regimen resulted not only in moderate weight loss but as high as a 30 percent decrease in knee pain, and as much as a 24 percent increase in knee function.

Here are some suggestions:

- Foods that contain sulfur, such as garlic, onion and eggs, can help repair and rebuild bone, cartilage and connective tissue, and also aid in absorbing calcium. Also, eat plenty of green leafy vegetables and other bright-colored vegetables, and non-acidic fresh fruit. Apples, blueberries and other berries, for example, would be better for arthritis sufferers than citrus fruits. Fresh pineapple in particular – not dried or canned – is very good because it has the enzyme bromelain, which can help reduce inflammation.

- Staying on a diet low in saturated fat when you have arthritis is important because this unhealthy fat leads to the development of inflammatory substances. But eat a lot of oily fish, such as herring, sardines and salmon, because omega-3 oils have been proven to provide therapeutic benefits for arthritis. And cod liver oil, considered the cure-all and preventative for just about every ailment years ago, apparently does work, after all. Results in 2004 from a study at Cardiff University in Wales showed an average 86 percent reduction of the enzymes implicated in osteoarthritis in participants who were given a small dose of cod-liver oil every day.

- Some researchers have suggested avoiding the following foods when possible, or at least eating less of them: red meat, table salt, refined carbohydrates, fried foods, and cow's milk, cheese and other dairy products from cows because these foods have been implicated in inflammatory processes. As you can see, a lot of these foods aren't very healthy anyway. Goat milk or yogurt is probably OK, however, as are rice and soy products.

- Some physicians advocate avoiding members of the nightshade family of vegetables (peppers, paprika, eggplant, tomatoes and potatoes) because the solanine found in these foods can cause pain for some people. Unfortunately, some of these foods also have many healthy attributes, so it's important for people with osteoarthritis to find other good sources of the nutrients they may lose if they eliminate these foods from their diet. It's also a good idea to stay away from stimulants and depressants such as caffeine and alcohol.

- It's OK to get iron from food such as broccoli but make sure your nutritional supplements don't have extra iron unless you're anemic. There is some evidence that iron may be involved in the pain, swelling and even joint destruction of osteoarthritis.

In reviewing this list, it seems pretty obvious to me that so many aspects of a good and healthy diet, except perhaps for a few vegetables and fruits, may well be of benefit to osteoarthritis sufferers.

Prostate Problems

As men grow older, many develop prostrate problems, the most serious being prostate cancer. The other common problems are inflammation and prostate enlargement, which may block urine flow, making it weaker, slower and more frequent. These changes in the prostate don't necessarily indicate cancer by any means, but it's a good idea to get a PSA test for prostate cancer if they occur. A normal PSA count is 4 or less; mine is 1.6. A few nutritional supplements, primarily saw palmetto, have been recommended to help with these less serious problems. Reducing obesity, however, may help the most.

Modern research indicates that obesity, which figures prominently in so many serious diseases, is also a negative factor not only in prostate-cancer death rates but also the development of prostate disease.

One study compared the mortality rate from prostate cancer of men in Japan and the United States. They showed that five times more U.S. men die from prostate cancer than their counterparts in Japan. In fact, the frequency and the mortality rates of prostate cancer are significantly higher in the United States when compared with those in most Asian countries. Next to skin cancer, prostate cancer is the second-most-common cancer in men in this country.

The research looked at the diets of American men and found that the average American diet is about 40 percent fat, while the typical Japanese diet is only 10 percent to 20 percent fat. The Asian diet usually includes a lot of fish and many plant-based foods such as soy, fruits, vegetables and whole grains. The typical American diet has much larger amounts of processed foods and animal products, the main nutritional causes of obesity.

Earlier studies had shown that overall fat intake has a direct bearing on the incidence of prostate cancer, which increased in the 20th century in Western countries right along with the increase in the high-in-saturated-fat diets of red meat and desserts such as ice cream, and the hidden trans fat in foods like solid margarine and commercially baked goods.

In addition, two studies of obese prostate cancer patients showed their cancers were much more aggressive and more resistant to treatment than most. Both studies indicate that maintaining normal weight throughout your lifetime reduces your risk of developing more aggressive prostate cancer. The cancers were also much more likely to reoccur in obese men than in men who had maintained a healthy weight.

The best explanation is that obesity causes changes in the levels of reproductive hormones such as testosterone and estrogen, and of proteins such as leptin, an insulin-like growth factor, which are involved in cell growth and division. So reduction in the level of hormones like testosterone may have a big impact on the progression of prostate cancer.

One study showed testosterone levels to be quite a bit lower in middle-aged men who ate a lot of dietary fiber from cereals, grains, fruits and vegetables than in men eating a typical American diet filled with processed foods, and hence a much lower fiber content.

So eating a diet low in saturated fat and trans fat, and high in fiber, coupled with regular exercise, can help reduce the risk of prostate cancer by helping to prevent or reverse obesity, and by helping to reduce the aggressiveness of prostate cancer when it does occur.

But that's only part of what men can do to help reduce their prostate cancer risks. As you know by now, a growing amount of research indicates that fruits and vegetables have certain compounds and nutrients, such as vitamins A and C, that help the body destroy cancer-causing agents before they have a chance to damage cells. The best sources of these vitamins are dark green leafy vegetables such as spinach and romaine lettuce; red, orange or yellow vegetables such as carrots, sweet potatoes and red and yellow peppers; and citrus including oranges and grapefruit.

These colorful fruits and vegetables are also rich in plant chemicals (phytochemicals) that are now undergoing a great deal of research. In fact, it has already been shown in several studies that lycopene, the potent phytochemical prevalent in many red-colored vegetables and fruits, can keep prostate cancer tumors from growing and, in some instances, actually reduce the size of tumors.

In a well-known six-year Harvard University study of 47,000 middle-aged men who ate 10 servings of tomatoes a week — mostly from spaghetti sauce, although sometimes from pizza and other sources — cut their risk of prostate cancer by 45 percent. Men who ate four to seven servings weekly reduced the risk by 20 percent. The results reflected the lower rate of the cancer in southern Mediterranean men from countries such as Italy and Greece where tomato-based foods are a dietary staple. Cooking tomatoes in oil seemed to provide the most benefit.

Meanwhile, garlic, onions, shallots and leeks contain ganosulfur, compounds that have been shown in some laboratory studies to prevent tumor cell growth. These phytochemicals are best absorbed with a little cooking or crushing, which helps to release more of their benefits. And members of another family of vegetables called the cruciferous vegetables (including broccoli, cauliflower and Brussels sprouts) contain indoles, substances that also seem to block carcinogens from body cells.

Some researchers believe the difference in the incidence of — and the slower progression of — prostate cancer in countries like Japan could have to do with the soy-based foods in the traditional Asian diet. Recent studies have looked at the properties of phytochemicals called isoflavones — found only in soy — that may counteract the development of hormone-sensitive tumors like those in prostate cancer. Additionally, the isoflavone genestein has been shown in laboratory studies to inhibit the growth of both hormone-dependent as well as hormone-independent prostate cancer cells.

121

NUTRITION CONCERNS
FOR SENIORS

There is a genetic component to prostate cancer. But interestingly enough, a five-year collaboration between Japanese and American urological scientists yielded results in 2004 showing that Japanese men born and living in America had a four times higher rate of prostate cancer than Japanese men living in Japan. This was attributed to the differences between the Asian diet, high in soy and low in saturated fat, and the Western diet. Not incidentally, prostate cancer rates have risen in men in those Japanese cities where American fast-food eateries and their counterparts abound and where many work in sedentary jobs.

Although soy foods seem strange to many Americans, they can be made quite tasty and can be found in most supermarkets in various forms. Soybeans are actually legumes with a nutty flavor and can be used in any recipe that requires beans. Low-fat soymilk fortified with calcium and vitamin D is a healthy substitute for cow's whole milk and can be used the same way ordinary milk can, such as on cereals and in some recipes.

Some soy products, like tofu (bean curd) and textured vegetable (soy) protein, don't have much taste by themselves. However, added to various other foods they assume the flavors of what is in the mix. They also are a good substitute for meat in many recipes, such as hamburger or meatballs, and can be added to well-seasoned soups, stir-fries and stews. Soft or "silken" tofu works well in creamy dishes such as soups, dips and salad dressings.

Zinc may be another factor in good prostate health, because the healthy prostate normally has a fairly high concentration of zinc. So a diet too low in zinc could be a good predictor of future prostate disease. Sources of zinc include sesame, pumpkin and sunflower seeds; most nuts, and legumes like green peas; the outer coating of whole grains; spinach and to a lesser degree other leafy green vegetables; and tofu and mushrooms.

Once again, a healthy diet, in this case along with a focus on particular foods, may well decrease the risks of a major disease.

Other Factors of Concern for Seniors

Many of the problems leading to poor nutrition among seniors have to do with factors other than food choices. Some could be solved with better eating habits and exercise along with other lifestyle changes. But some seniors are very resistant to making these changes. And some poor nutrition in seniors has to do with conditions that are difficult to control.

122

NUTRITION CONCERNS
FOR SENIORS

For example, some of the seniors I know feel they are healthy enough now and don't want to change their eating habits or, for that matter, do much else that might help them lead a healthier life either now or in the future. Their argument is that they've worked hard and now want to enjoy life, even if it takes years off that life. They just don't want to hear about a way of eating that doesn't sound like much fun. And they don't think change will help them anyway because it's too late. I think you know by now how I feel about that.

I think it's true some seniors just don't have the information they need about good nutrition or even realize they need to have this information. Among my reasons for writing this book is to make this information available in a way that is pertinent to seniors. I hope to show you how to make healthy changes and to see that it is possible to be as old as I am and still be in good health and living an active and fulfilling life.

Older people can be prone to certain circumstances, in their lifestyle, besides overeating and not wanting to change their lifestyle, that can negatively affect nutrition. They may, for example, have lost their spouse and friends of many years. With no one there to share a meal, they may revert to unhealthy foods for dinner.

Some seniors have lost much of their sense of smell as they have aged, and consequently also some of their sense of taste. Since food no long tastes as good as it once did, they haven't much interest in it and eat only out of habit whatever happens to be handy. Or they find they have no appetite anymore and so eat very little.

Perhaps, like many senior men, you've never cooked a meal in your life and don't think you can. Or maybe you are generally healthy but have experienced a loss of eyesight, leading to problems in the kitchen with cooking and preparing food. Also, seniors who can't see as well as they used to and don't drive much may be reticent to ask others to take them to shop for food. The small groceries that used to deliver hardly exist anymore, and when they do, the food is usually more expensive than it is at the regular supermarket. Self-sufficient all their lives, these folks now may make do with what is in the cupboard for as long as they can.

What many seniors, even those on fixed incomes, don't realize is that it doesn't cost any more to eat healthy foods than it does to eat unhealthy foods; in fact, it might cost less. It just takes time and planning.

If you are a senior with some of these difficulties, there is help out

NUTRITION CONCERNS
FOR SENIORS

there for you. Do what you can for yourself – invite friends or family to share a meal, for example – but don't be afraid or embarrassed to ask for help. You might be surprised to find how people with altruistic natures want to help. They enjoy helping others and have the ability to do it. Sometimes that can help them as much as it can help you. It makes them feel good about themselves and gives them a sense of accomplishment and purpose.

In addition, there are probably a number of government or non-profit organizations in your community that offer services for seniors, some staffed mainly by volunteers. While it is beyond the scope of this book to directly connect you with this sort of assistance, we do provide telephone numbers and e-mail addresses of national offices of organizations that may be able to assist you to find the help you need locally. These can be found in the back of the book under Services for Seniors.

CHAPTER 15

THE DOS AND DON'TS IN YOUR NUTRITIONAL PLAN

- Do avoid food with unhealthy saturated fats and trans fat. Do choose sources of healthy unsaturated fats, such as canola and olive oils, and of healthy omega-3 fatty acids, such as salmon and nuts.

- In general, do avoid "white" foods, such as white potatoes, white rice, white flour, white bread, white pasta, sugar and salt. Exceptions are garlic, onion and cauliflower.

- Do learn how to shop healthy. Don't skip reading the labels on cans and packages of food. Familiarize yourself with how to read them and judge for yourself if it's a good choice for you. Don't purchase any food product unless you are thoroughly familiar with its nutritional content.

- Do include as many fruits and vegetables as possible in your diet. Usually, the darker and more vivid the color, the more nutritious the food.

- Do avoid cleaning your plate, especially when the serving is larger than necessary. It's better to leave extra food on your plate than in your stomach. Be especially careful when eating away from home.

- Don't let yourself get too hungry or you may end up overeating. Learn how to make healthy snacks and take them with you whenever you can. Snacking as many as three times a day is fine, as long you're eating healthy foods.

- Don't fix yourself a healthy salad and smother it with an unhealthy dressing that's high in saturated fat. And don't top a healthy dish of fresh blueberries with two scoops of ice cream. Fortunately, there is now a wide assortment of healthier choices available, such as non-fat salad dressings and fat-free, sugar-free toppings.

- Don't neglect your fiber. As senior citizens, we need a little more than we used to. Raw vegetables, fruits, legumes and whole-grain (unrefined) products such as brown rice and whole-wheat bread provide adequate daily fiber needs.

- Don't be fooled by the terms "low-fat," "lower-fat" or "reduced fat." Take the time to learn how to interpret what these actually mean. Foods with these labels may have more fat, especially saturated fat or trans-fat (usually listed as "partially hydrogenated" oils), than you bargained for. Also, many of these products – even non-fat ones – are loaded with sodium and/or sugar or sweeteners like honey.

- If possible, don't keep anything in the house on a regular basis that would prove to be a temptation if it's not in your best dietary interest.

PART II
EXERCISE

CHAPTER 16

WHY NOT START EXERCISING RIGHT NOW?

Talk to any physician or health expert and you'll hear the same thing: exercise is critical to good health. Nothing you can do will replace the positive effects on your health that come from exercise. Perhaps that's not the greatest revelation, but too often we think aging and exercise don't mix. The opposite is true. Everyone needs to exercise – especially those of us over 65 – even if it means just going for a lively walk or taking a relaxing swim.

When I speak about health, there are always those in the audience who are taken aback when they hear that I go to a gym and work out on weight machines every day even though I'm in my 80s. I explain that my workout, though vigorous, is tailored for me and for what I can do. As you read this section you'll get a firsthand look at the "Seretean Routine" that was designed specifically for me. There is no way I can do the same regimen as a healthy and strong 20-, 40- or even 50-year-old can. But that's not the point. The point of exercising is to keep your body running smoothly. And even a few minutes sitting in a chair and lifting your legs or moving your arms can make a difference.

Just for a minute, let's look at the human body like an automobile. To keep your car running well, you need to make sure it has fuel for energy and oil to keep the moving parts from wearing out, and you need to get it up and running frequently so parts don't rust or deteriorate.

The same is true for your body. In the body, the fuel is food. And just like in a car, the better the quality of the fuel, the better the body will run. You wouldn't expect your car to run well on dirty or diluted fuel, so why would you expect your body not to sputter when you fill it with foods full of saturated fats or with processed ingredients?

Would you expect your car to run without oil to keep the parts well lubricated and the engine purring? Of course not. But too many people forget to drink enough fluids to keep all the parts working properly. And most of us know that in order for your car to function properly when you want it to, you have to use it. If you don't, the battery dies, the oil leaks and the hoses dry out and crack. It simply won't function when you want it to if you don't use it often enough.

Take it for a spin every day and it's quite a different story. The oil is flowing, the pistons are pumping and everything is working smoothly. Take care of that car and it will last for many years. Don't take care of it, and it can be in poor condition after just 15,000 to 20,000 miles. The same holds true for your body.

I'm sure there will be days when you don't feel like taking the car for a spin, when you'd rather stay in bed or don't want to have to face foul weather. But in the end, you know the car will run better and will be more dependable if you do what needs to be done.

The same holds true with exercise. There are days when getting up and going to the gym is the last thing I want to do. But on those days when I drag myself into the gym to work out, I discover that exercise makes a difference. Within six or seven minutes of getting started, I'm feeling much better physically and mentally and I have a little bounce in my step. For me, there's great pleasure at the end of the exercises – pleasure in knowing I've done it and that I'm keeping my body healthy. I also get pleasure in knowing I've just earned my next meal. Each of us has our own reasons to exercise and each of us can make up our own excuses.

For me, knowing I'm in better shape than I was 10 years ago, or even 25 years ago, keeps me going. What inspires me is the possibility that I might be in better shape 10 years from now at age 90. Who knows? But I'm going to give it my best shot. And I also enjoy looking and feeling good – something that definitely comes from getting the proper amount of exercise. What I've discovered for myself is that every day can be more fruitful if you look and feel better. It's a perennial upper!

As we go through this chapter, we'll talk about a few ways to keep yourself motivated during your exercises, We'll talk about fun ways to get the exercise you need and about making sure the exercise you're doing is right for you. You'll also discover, in this section of the book, that you can take small steps – literally and figuratively – that will make a big difference. During the course of any given day, each of us has a chance to make a difference in the length and health of our lives through simple decisions. There are so many ways to exercise, so many enjoyable things you can do that will make you feel better.

Why not start exercising and start right now?

CHAPTER 17

THE BENEFITS OF EXERCISE

Exercise is an integral part of my daily routine. Chances are that if I don't make it to the community gym for my 50-minute aerobic weight-training daily regimen, I do a reduced version on my mini-gym at home or walk three miles around my community.

You might ask, "Does someone in his 70s or 80s really need to exercise?"

You do if you want to live a long and healthy life. There's plenty of scientific data that shows exercise is good for your heart and helps your body stave off serious diseases. According to the President's Council on Physical Fitness, there are 300,000 preventable deaths each year in which physical inactivity is a contributing factor. A sedentary lifestyle is one of the major risk factors for several diseases, especially heart disease and cancer, that can reduce your quality of life.

Research used by the President's Council, which came from reports published by government agencies such as the Department of Health and Human Services and the Surgeon General's Office, strongly supports the belief that a moderate amount of exercise provides significant health benefits. It also shows that greater amounts of physical activity can lead to additional benefits. Yet, according to the research, about 40 percent of Americans say they don't exercise at all, while seven out of 10 Americans say they don't receive the 30 minutes of moderate activity five days a week recommended by the medical and scientific communities.

If you're one of those people, it's not too late to consider making a change in your lifestyle, because if you're not getting any exercise you're taking a risk with your health – not just your physical health, but your mental health as well. One of my goals in this section of the book is to show you how easy it is to make that change and to provide you with specific exercises and activities that will help you get the most out of your physical activity. I'll also tell you about some of the equipment you might want to buy and about ways to keep motivated while you're working out.

Researchers have found the greatest obstacles standing in the way of people getting physical activity are time, access to convenient facilities, and safe environments in which to be active. As you read on, you'll see that all you really need is 30 minutes and you can get the exercise you need without ever having to leave your home.

Unless you live in a cocoon, you know exercise is critical to helping you control your weight and reduce your body fat. But did you know scientists have good reason to believe exercise will reduce your risk of dying from Type 2 diabetes, cardiovascular disease and certain cancers, such as colon cancer?

In the United States, cardiovascular disease, which leads to strokes and heart attacks, is the leading cause of death among both men and women, and people who are physically inactive are more at risk of developing it. Doctors will tell you physical inactivity ranks right up there with cigarette smoking and high blood pressure as a risk factor for cardiovascular disease. Yet it's among the easiest risk factors to control.

There's scientific evidence, according to the President's Council, that daily physical activity can help you lower your blood pressure and cholesterol, can help prevent or slow down the development of osteoporosis, and can reduce the symptoms of arthritis. There is also a strong belief, based on scientific studies, that exercise can help reduce anxiety and depression. For most people, exercise is a great stress reliever – a chance to focus on a workout and not your worries – and plays a large role in mental and physical wellness. Exercise can also help you get a better night's sleep, and that helps you feel better throughout the day.

Before I go too much further here, I want to make sure we're clear on one thing. You don't have to go out and sign up to work out at the local gym in order to get the exercise you need. You'll see in this section of the book that you can get a good workout just by taking a walk, going out dancing or riding a bike. In this section, I also introduce you to exercises you can do at home without having to buy any extra equipment.

You're not ready to start doing push-ups and crunches? Well, you don't have to start with the tough stuff. As you'll see, the best way to do any of these exercises is to ease your way into them. Remember, however, to check with your doctor before starting any exercise program.

Once you do start getting a significant amount of exercise, you're more than likely to find that your weight will start going down, especially if you eat healthfully. That's important, especially when you consider

THE BENEFITS OF EXERCISE

that more than 60 percent of adults in the United States are overweight, according to government statistics. You might also find that some of those aches and pains start to go away and that working around the house becomes easier. As you develop your back muscles, for example, you're helping to prevent back pain. Develop your biceps and triceps as well as your shoulder muscles and you have less trouble lifting the groceries.

Here are two more great benefits to exercising: you look a lot better and you get to save a few bucks you might be spending right now on doctor bills or medicines. It's estimated, according to the federal government, that it costs more than $117 billion each year in medical expenses just for the treatment and care of people who are overweight.

CHAPTER 18

WALKING FOR YOUR HEALTH

Do you get annoyed when you just miss that parking spot next to the grocery store and end up having to hike a few hundred yards to do your shopping?

Do you find yourself wishing the elevator to the second floor would get there a lot more quickly but never consider climbing the steps?

Do you prefer to wait to get on a crowded escalator at the airport or stadium rather than walk up the ramp?

If the answer is yes to all of these, then you're missing a great opportunity to partake in one of the simplest and most effective forms of exercise: walking.

There's no doubt a good brisk walk every day provides you with the daily exercise you need to stay healthy. And studies show it's never too late to start. Researchers who studied 9,500 women over 65 during a 13-year period discovered that women who started walking a mile a day were less likely to die from heart disease or cancer than women who didn't exercise. The study found that the active women had a 40 percent to 50 percent lower risk of dying from these diseases than their sedentary counterparts.

Does this mean you should go out and start walking a mile tomorrow? Of course not. What it does mean is you should consider taking a walk every day, even if it's a short walk. You'll find the walk can be relaxing and help you relieve stress. It is also an exercise you can do with someone else. And you can just about always find a place to walk, whether it's in your neighborhood or at the local mall.

It is widely believed a 35-minute brisk walk three or four days a week gives you the minimum amount of aerobic exercise you need. But if you really want to get serious about staying healthy, then you might want to walk for 35 minutes or more *every* day. On the flip side, you might not be ready for even a 35-minute walk, so start with a shorter one. As I've said before, any kind of walking is good, but the more energetic the walk, the more you get out of it.

How do you know if you're walking fast enough to get the most out of your exercise? One way is to measure your heart rate to see if it's up between 100 and 120 beats a minute. Another way to know if you're on the right track is to see if you can work up a light sweat, more of a sheen, by the time you're finished.

Once you've determined you're going to walk, you'll have to figure out where and when. One of the most convenient places to walk is in your own neighborhood. Having traveled quite a bit, I've discovered that just about every neighborhood has places where you can walk safely.

But if you do walk in the neighborhood, you'll want to take some precautions. If you walk at night and you're in an area with no sidewalks, make sure approaching traffic can see you. Wear light-colored clothing, carry a flashlight or wear reflective material, and walk in a secure, well-lighted area. If you walk during the day, don't forget to apply sun block. If you're exercising outside, try to walk on even surfaces, whether they're paved or unpaved, so you don't lose your balance. It's also good to find scenic routes or walk with a friend so you can stay interested.

Some researchers believe if you do walk outside, you might consider doing so in an area with hills or steps in order to get even more out of the workout. But one of the best places to walk, I believe, is at a shopping mall. Obviously, you don't have to worry about weather or cars and you can also do quite a bit of sightseeing as you make your way from one end to the other. That helps you keep your mind off the fact that you're exercising and helps you avoid boredom. What you discover is by the time you've gone from one end of the mall to the other a couple of times, you've logged a few miles.

And don't forget the treadmill. You can always log a few miles this way if you have one at your home or at the gym. Once again, you're indoors in a controlled environment, so you need not worry about traffic or weather. You might, however, have to fight off boredom, something we'll address in a minute.

When is the best time to walk? Some people choose the mornings, but I believe you get the most out of walking in the evenings, preferably after dinner. Walking helps you bring up your metabolic rate, which normally slows after around 7:30 p.m. Increasing your metabolism helps you avoid that sluggish feeling and can keep you active. Walking in the evening can also help you avoid craving a late-night snack because it depresses your appetite to some degree.

WALKING FOR YOUR HEALTH

For me, one of the best reasons to walk in the evening is that light exercise at that time of day can induce relaxation and a good night's sleep. As we get older, we often find sleeping through the night to be a challenge.

For some, the best way to avoid getting bored when they walk is to share the activity with a partner and maintain a steady conversation. I prefer to wear a headset and listen to good music. And when I do exercise on a treadmill, I'm sure to have my headset on or the television or both so I can take my mind off the exercise.

I often see people hoping to enhance their exercise by adding weights to their walk. But some physiologists believe wearing or carrying weights can do more harm than good if it's not done properly. Many believe belts or vests with pockets provide the best way to add weights because the weight is evenly distributed. Another idea is to wear a backpack with books or other weighty items, as long as the weight is evenly distributed.

Some of you might say, "I just don't have time to walk." But the truth is, everyone can make walking a part of his or her daily ritual. The next time you're looking for a parking spot at the mall, find a safe area a little farther away. You'll enjoy the walk and won't be nearly as stressed about getting the perfect spot before the next car comes along.

CHAPTER 19

JUST DANCE

Exercise doesn't have to be boring or dull. It doesn't even have to be overly strenuous. Sometimes you'll be getting a great workout doing something you really enjoy – and you might not even know it.

One of the best exercise activities for people 55 and up is dancing. Just think about it for a minute. You're indoors, having fun with a partner while going pretty much at your own pace. You can sit out a dance if you're too tired or you can dance the whole night away. It's great aerobic exercise, and anyone can do it as long as you're physically able to stand. Best of all, dancing is fun and not work.

What makes dancing the perfect exercise is its simplicity and accessibility. Chances are that no matter where you live, you'll find a dance club, dance hall, community center, or school dancing facilities near you. Lessons are usually available at all of these locations. And in most of the places you'll find instructors teaching every conceivable dance step from rock to Latin to the Foxtrot.

Often community centers or schools offer dance classes at a very reasonable price, and my guess is that if there's enough interest, it would be easy to get a program started near you if one isn't available. The truth is almost anyone can be a dancer, even if you have two left feet. And you'll discover that age is no barrier. Even now, in my 80s, I enjoy going to a local ballroom to dance. It's one of my favorite activities and it's very reasonably priced at $9 per person. One gets a fairly healthy sandwich and beverage and the opportunity to dance from 5 to 11 p.m. on a huge dance floor with some of the very best dancers in Florida.

One couple in particular, who go every week to this same local ballroom, is fascinating to watch. The woman, who must be in her mid-80s, and her husband, who must be in his 90s, dance non-stop. They move beautifully to the beat and are an inspiration for other, much younger dancers. It's not only a great place for couples, it's also a great place for singles since, generally speaking, anyone can dance with anyone else.

What makes dancing great exercise? Well, for the most part, your arms and legs are in constant motion while you're on the dance floor. Essentially what you're doing is walking quickly, and we've already established the benefits of a brisk walk. Spend three or four hours dancing and you'll probably end up covering two or three miles.

Another benefit to dancing is that it helps you with your sense of balance, which might not be as strong as it was in years past. Because you're working with a partner, and in many cases holding onto a partner, you can feel more secure. In many ways dancing also can help to enhance your coordination.

Dancing isn't just good physical exercise, it's mental exercise as well. You're constantly thinking. You have to stay with the rhythm and at the same time you're thinking about challenges such as changing direction or innovating with different steps.

There are, of course, some dances that are more strenuous than others and provide more of a workout. Tap dancing is an example of a dance that requires one to be in good physical shape. I know from firsthand experience.

After I turned 70, I decided to do some things I always wanted to do. I had grown up watching the likes of Fred Astaire, Dan Dailey, Gene Kelly, and Donald O'Connor – the best-known tap dancers of that era. I wanted to add my name to that list (just kidding). I found a tap-dancing instructor who was willing to teach me in my home. For seven months, I took three one-hour tap-dancing lessons each week. With every lesson, I sweated bullets and lost between a pound-and-a-half and two pounds. It was very strong aerobic exercise – flexibility, balance and mental exertion packaged together.

I was frankly relieved when the lessons ended. My teacher and I then taped our three big numbers and I rested on my laurels. I don't believe I threatened the best of today's tap dancers, but nevertheless I feel it was one of my proudest accomplishments considering my age.

Not too long ago, there was a popular song called "I Hope You Dance" about the importance of living life to its fullest and making sure you experience all it has to offer. In the chorus, country singer Lee Ann Womack tells her listeners she hopes they'll dance through life rather than sit it out on the sidelines.

That goes for me, too – probably for different reasons, but I hope if you have the chance to either sit it out or dance, that you'll dance. In the long run, you'll be glad you did.

CHAPTER 20

OTHER AEROBIC EXERCISES

Just about any exercise is good for you if you work up a mild sweat and get to the point where you're breathing hard but not out of breath. Among the many choices are programs you'll find at a health club or gym, such as aerobics and spinning classes, as well as sports such as tennis, golf or even senior softball, which is popular here in Florida.

Along with walking, two of the best aerobic exercises for those of us over 55, however, may be swimming and bicycling.

Why? Well, both offer you a chance to increase your endurance and they're good at strengthening muscles. In short, swimming and bicycling offer you a chance to do exercises that help you every day. Let's talk about each one.

Swimming

One of the best things about swimming, especially for people in our age bracket, is that it's a low-impact exercise. Because we're in the water and we have our natural buoyancy working for us, our muscles and bones don't tend to get the jarring impact that can come with jogging, tennis or other weight-bearing exercises or sports.

Swimming is also more gentle on our joints. You hardly ever hear of swimmers suffering from the serious knee or shoulder injuries associated with other sports. If you suffer from arthritis or back problems, or if you just don't like jarring your body, swimming might be the perfect exercise for you since it's unlikely to have a negative impact on your body.

At the same time, however, swimming provides the resistance we need to make our muscles work better. And one of the best-known effects of swimming is that it involves most of our muscle groups. Varying your strokes can help ensure you get the most out of swimming. The backstroke, for example, works different sets of muscles than the typical crawl. Generally speaking, swimming works all of your muscles, from your abs and quads to your triceps and biceps. Another great thing about swimming is that it's a good way to burn up the calories while keeping your joints flexible. In swimming, the movement of your head in and out of the water can help keep your neck limber while your shoulders and hips also get a great workout. Swimming, some believe, is especially good for seniors because it helps us develop our coordination, which in turn can help reduce the risk of falls.

So what's the best way to get the most out of your swimming exercise? We recommend you warm up and stretch first before starting, and some simple stretches to loosen your back and your neck are always good. It's also a good idea to stretch out your shoulders and your legs.

Warming up can take many forms. You might just want to walk around the pool a couple of times at a pretty steady rate to get your heart going, or you may want to slowly paddle around in the pool before you get down to serious exercise. It's good to spend about five or 10 minutes warming up.

Once you're ready, you should swim for 20 to 40 minutes, usually continuous laps, using different strokes. Going to the pool three or four times a week can help you build up your endurance and lose some pounds as well. Of course, you're going to want to start off slowly and build up to a serious workout.

It's important to note that while swimming might be good for your joints and muscles, it's not an exercise that will strengthen your bones. And of course, if you're going to embark on a swim program, make sure you're in a safe environment with a phone or another person nearby to help in an emergency.

You might also want to consider some other programs, including water aerobics, which are offered at many community centers and swim clubs.

Bicycling

Many of us grew up riding bicycles as our primary mode of transportation. But as we got older, we traded in our handlebars for steering wheels. Now might be a good time to do just the opposite.

If you're planning to visit a neighbor or make a trip to the store a few blocks away, why not keep the car in the garage and pull out the bicycle instead? Or perhaps you might just want to take the bike for a ride through the neighborhood after dinner.

You'll find that bicycling is not only a great aerobic exercise, it's also a good way to build up your balance and really strengthen your leg muscles. Why is that so important? As you'll read later in the book, one of the biggest obstacles to reaching our goal of living to 100 is the common fall. If we take steps to improve our balance and strengthen our leg muscles, chances of falling and injuring our knees or hips can be reduced.

In addition to helping your muscles, a bike ride is good for your heart and your lungs. It's also good for helping you lose weight. It's estimated that riding a bike for about an hour will burn about 300 calories, as long as you're riding at a pace that increases your heart rate. Again, a good barometer of how much you're getting out of the exercise will be if you're breathing heavily but are not out of breath.

As you'll see later in this section, I spend about 15 minutes every day on the stationary bike at my gym. Of course, for me the bike is just one part of my daily routine, so I don't need to spend an hour riding. But if you're not participating in other exercises, biking for an hour a day, three or four days a week, could be very beneficial.

Should you decide to bicycle outdoors, I strongly recommend you wear a bicycle helmet and take other safety precautions, including bringing a cell phone with you, just to be on the safe side.

Aerobic exercises can be fun and can build up your endurance while at the same time strengthening your heart, your lungs and your muscles.

CHAPTER 21

THE BIG STRETCH

Stretching is one of the most important things you can do before beginning exercises, whether you're just going for a walk or are hitting the weight-lifting machines.

The reason is simple. Stretching helps to loosen your muscles so when you do exercise, you can reduce the risk of injury and increase flexibility and mobility.

Animals know this instinctively. The first thing my cat does when he gets up from a nap is stretch out his front and back legs. Dogs also do this, as do most other animals. People can benefit from stretching as soon as they get up in the morning, especially as they get older. Exercise physiologists believe stretching can significantly counteract the shortening that naturally occurs in our muscles, ligaments and tendons as our bodies and skeletal structures age. This process can limit flexibility. But it doesn't have to.

Before you get too deep into the day, try lying flat on your back with your feet straight out and pull your arms straight back over your head. You'll feel your abdomen muscles stretch and you'll also feel it in your shoulders, back and arms. Stretch like that for about 10 to 15 seconds and you'll be better prepared for the day. As I've frequently mentioned, it's never too late to start exercising, and that goes for stretching as well.

According to the National Institute on Aging, it's always best to warm up before you begin your stretches. If you're just planning to do stretches, then you might want to do a little walking first or perhaps do light exercises. Stretching without warming up first could result in injury. There are books available and there's information online that can help you with some light exercises to do before stretching. And if you plan on doing any weight lifting, it's essential you stretch your muscles before beginning a workout, in order to reduce the risk of injuries.

If you go to a gym, you might see some people who stretch after every exercise. While that's a good thing, it's not absolutely necessary, but stretching muscles before putting them to the test is something that can help prevent serious injury.

You'll want to do each stretch three to five times, according to the Institute on Aging, and hold each stretch for 10 to 30 seconds. Stretch the muscles as far as you can. You should feel mild discomfort but never pain. This is called static stretching. Make your efforts smooth. A jerky or bouncy motion during stretching can lead to injury.

One way to get the best out of stretches is to go through a full rotation, working on each muscle, and then repeat the entire series. If you're going to do strength training, it's best to warm up for 10 minutes, stretch for 10 minutes, lift for 30 minutes, then stretch again. Stretching after strength training helps loosen tight muscles and promotes recuperation.

Here are nine other stretches that can help to loosen your muscles before you try any heavy exercise or lifting.

Wall Push

In this stretch, put your hands straight out in front with your palms against a wall. Place one leg in front of the other and push forward with the back leg. Hold for 15 seconds. You'll feel the stretching in your calves, hamstrings and buttocks. Make sure to stretch both legs.

Shoulder Stretch

Stand with one arm extended out and bent at the elbow at a 90-degree angle so you look as if you're about to be sworn in at a court hearing. Now put your palm against a wall or doorjamb and rotate your body away from the wall. Hold for 15 seconds. You'll feel the tugging on the muscles in your shoulders.

Triceps Stretch

Put your right arm behind your head, forearm bent at the elbow, so your hand is touching the middle of your back. With your left hand, grab your right elbow and pull it to the left so you're stretching the triceps. Hold for 15 seconds. Then change arms.

Pec Stretch

Put your right arm in front of your chest, with your right hand resting on your left shoulder. With your left hand, grab your elbow and pull your arm up so you feel the stretching in your right pectoral muscle. Hold for 15 seconds. You'll also feel it in your back. Then change hands.

Back Stretch

Place your right hand against a wall in front of you, waist high, and push your right leg forward. Push and twist your body slightly to the left and hold the stretch for 15 seconds before switching arms and legs.

Raised Leg Stretch

This is a stretch you can really feel in your hamstrings and thighs. Stand on one leg and raise the other forward, resting it on a chair or a high step. As you lean forward, you will feel more of a stretch. Hold it for 15 seconds and then change legs.

Toe Touches

This is as easy as standing straight up and then reaching down to touch your toes without bending your knees. Once again, you'll feel the muscles stretch in the back of your legs. Hold it for 15 seconds, then stretch again. For those just starting out, you might want to just wrap your hands as far down your legs as possible.

Thigh Stretch

Start by standing on your right foot and pulling your left foot behind your right leg with your right hand. This will help limber up your thigh muscles. Change legs and repeat the process.

Neck Stretch

It's easy to forget this one, but it can be important in loosening muscles in your neck and shoulders. Put your right arm over your head with your right hand on your left ear. Keeping your body straight, pull your head to the right so you can feel the muscles in your neck stretch. Then gently repeat with your left hand, stretching your neck to the left.

Remember, stretching before exercising will help minimize the risk of injury. Stretching before starting the day helps with mobility and flexibility, making it easier to do your daily tasks. And if you can't do other exercises for some reason, try stretching three times a week for at least 20 minutes.

For more stretches and other information, visit the National Institute on Aging's website at: http://www.weboflife.nasa.gov/exerciseandaging/home.html.

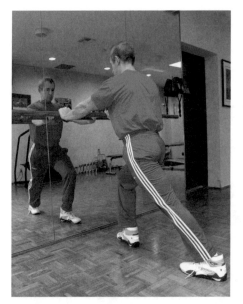

Wall Push

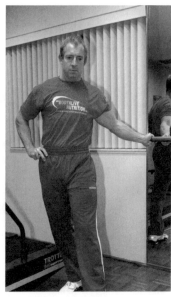

Shoulder Stretch

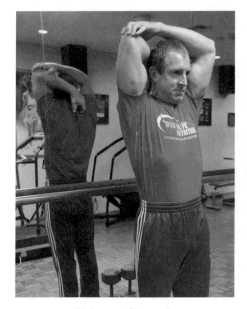

Triceps Stretch

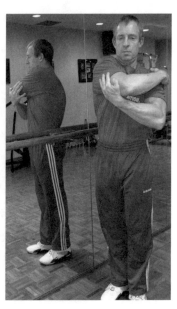

Pec Stretch

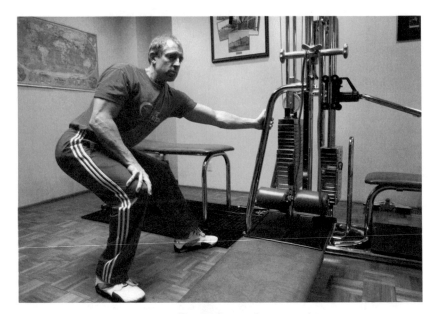

Back Stretch

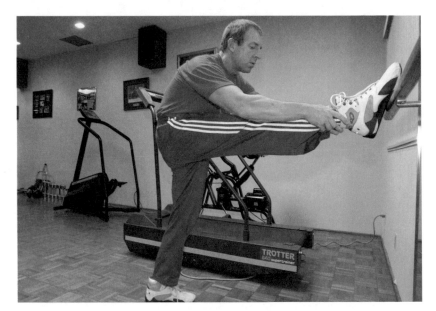

Raised Leg Stretch

146

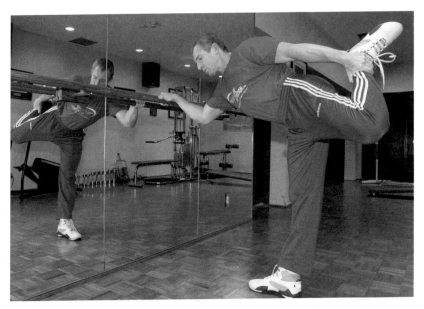

Thigh Stretch

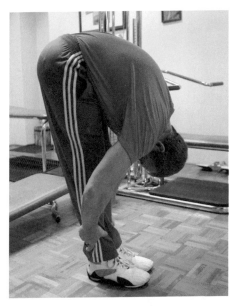

Toe Touches

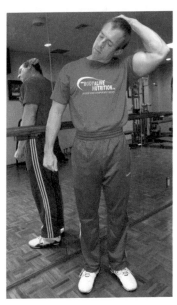

Neck Stretch

CHAPTER 22

STRENGTH TRAINING WITHOUT APPARATUS

If you want to get a good workout but you don't want to join a gym or buy expensive home fitness equipment, then this chapter is perfect for you. This chapter is also good for people who might need a little exercise when they're away from home and not near any fitness facilities.

With the help of Tom Baggott, former executive chef at the Pritikin Longevity Center and a lifelong body builder, I've put together 10 simple exercises you can do in your home without any equipment that will work just about every muscle in your body. All you need are a doorframe, two doorknobs and a set of steps. By doing these exercises on a regular basis, you can help minimize the risk of injury from falls, back and leg problems and even heart disease. You can also improve your ability to perform daily chores such as lifting and carrying the groceries, and you'll improve your agility as well. Perhaps the best part is you'll feel better, maybe look better, and more than likely boost your self-esteem.

As with all exercises, it's important to start at a level that's comfortable for you. And there are some you might want to skip until you're in better shape. But eventually, you should be able to work up to a point where you can do three sets of 10 to 20 repetitions. Remember, age should not be a deterrent to exercise.

Doorknob Isometric Curls

This exercise will help you build up your biceps and make it easier for you to lift objects in your home. To do this exercise, open a door and stand facing its side. Now put your hands under the doorknobs on either side and pull up. Hold it for five seconds, relax for five seconds and repeat the exercise.

Doorway Isometric Press

With the door still open, reach up and push hard against the overhead part of the doorframe. Once again, push for about five seconds before resting for five seconds. You'll begin to feel the muscles in your back and shoulders tighten and grow stronger. This exercise will help you in practical ways, such as when you're trying to reach objects on shelves.

Free Chest Press

Now close the door and face it. Put your arms out in front of you and push hard against the door for five seconds. You'll feel the pressure on muscles in your back and you'll also be strengthening your arms. While you're doing this exercise, remember to breathe in while pushing and breathe out during the relaxation.

Stairway Free Calf Raise

This exercise strengthens your calf muscles and ankles and can help you keep your legs strong. It works best on the bottom step of a flight of stairs but can also be done on a phone book pushed up against a wall. Holding a railing with one hand, stand on the bottom step with just your toes. Then let the rest of your foot hang down.

The Stair Climb

This is a great aerobic exercise that helps you build your leg muscles and improve your circulation. Start very slowly and build up your repetitions until you're spending a minimum of 20 minutes walking up and down stairs. This will give you a good cardiovascular workout and exercise your legs. Be sure to check with your doctor before doing this exercise.

Walking Lunges

This is an exercise that will help you improve your circulation and stretch your leg muscles. As you walk, lunge forward, bending one leg at the knee and stretching out the other leg. If this is too strenuous, you can always start with a half lunge or a quarter lunge and build your way up. This exercise will strengthen your buttocks and your back and provide aerobic exercise.

Free Squats

This is one of the best exercises you can find because it works most of your muscle groups and builds circulation in your legs. Done properly, free squats can help prevent back injury and also help you remain mobile.

To do a squat properly, stand straight up, then bend at the knees and bring your buttocks down to just above the floor before standing back up. Once again, if you don't feel comfortable starting off with full squats, you can start with quarter squats or half squats and work your way up.

Jumping Jacks

Jumping jacks not only improve your balance and agility but they can also help to strengthen your bones because they're weight-bearing exercises. As a result, you're less likely to fall and sustain an injury. As with most exercises, the beauty of jumping jacks is that you can start at any level and build. If you only feel comfortable starting off with sets of five, then go from there.

To do a jumping jack, stand at attention with your hands by your side. Then simply jump, spreading your legs apart and bringing your hands together above your head. Jump again and return to the starting position.

Push-Ups

Push-ups help build strength in your arms, shoulders and chest. But don't worry if you're not in good enough shape yet to do a push-up. You can always start with a modified push-up, which is done on your knees instead of your toes. Once you build your strength, you might want to start doing regular push-ups. Either way, you'll be building muscles you need for lifting things in your home.

Crunches

Strengthening your abdominal muscles is a great way to prevent back injury. Crunches are similar to sit-ups in that you put your hands behind your head, but with a crunch you're simply raising your body a few inches off the floor while contracting your abdominal muscles. With crunches, your legs should be bent while you lie flat on your back.

CHAPTER 23

STRENGTH TRAINING WITH BANDS

When most people think of resistance training, they envision a gymnasium filled with barbells and dumbbells. But you might not be ready to spend time and money going to the gym. And purchasing good-quality home exercise equipment could take a significant investment.

Fortunately, there's a set of exercises you can do to provide you with a full-body workout. And it won't cost an arm and a leg but will help you to make sure the arms and legs you've got, as well as most other parts of your body, look and feel stronger.

All you need is a small piece of equipment called resistance-training (or toning) tubes. These elastic bands, usually about 4 feet in length with handles on each end, cost from $10 to $15 and are manufactured by companies such as GoFit or Reebok. You can find them at just about any sporting goods or exercise store.

The beauty of exercise tubes is that you are, in most cases, using your own body to provide the resistance you need to strengthen your muscles. And while your prime objective isn't to be a Charles Atlas look-alike, you do want strong muscles so you're able to perform routine household chores and prevent back or bone injuries. With the help of Tom Baggott again, I've compiled a list of several exercises you can do with exercise tubes that is an easy and effective way to transition into the next level of exercise.

As you go through these exercises, remember one of the key philosophies of this section: don't go too far too fast. As always, you'll want to be able to comfortably do three sets of 15 repetitions before increasing the resistance. And throughout the workout you'll want to make sure you remember the proper breathing technique, exhaling as you do the strenuous part of the exercise.

Here's another word of caution: there are items advertised on television and in magazines that, while similar to the exercise tubes, may come with a heftier price tag or promises that can't be kept. Be wary of these offers and remember, somebody has to pay for those television commercials.

Squats

This exercise is perfect for building strong quadriceps and hamstring muscles and can be adapted to help strengthen the inner thighs and provide better muscle tone. To do this exercise, put the middle of the tube under your feet, with your feet together. Make sure the lengths of band in each hand are equal and make sure your arms are down by your side, with your forearms extended straight out in front of you at the elbow. Breathe in as you squat down and breathe out as you come up, feeling the resistance in your legs.

To add resistance, simply spread your feet apart slightly, in essence shortening the length of band in each hand. Also, to strengthen the inner thigh, push your feet out to the side like a duck and do the standard three sets of 15 repetitions.

Curls

Curls are designed to help you build your biceps, and that's especially important if you need to do any lifting. In this exercise, you want to once again stand on the tube so you have equal lengths in each hand. Your arms will be down at your side, bent at the elbow, with your hands extended out, palms upward. Bend your knees slightly, breathe in and then breathe out as you do a regular curl. Drop your hands down by your side and then pull up with your forearms out in front of you at a 90-degree angle. You should feel the resistance in your arms. Once again, you can increase the resistance by simply moving your legs farther apart.

Tricep Press

This exercise will help you strengthen the muscles on the bottom of your arms and give shape to your triceps, which can easily lose their tone. Again, you want to step on the tube and have equal lengths in each hand. This time you're going to put your hands behind your head, with your thumbs down, and pull straight up. It's important to have your knees slightly bent and your feet together until you're ready to increase resistance.

Lateral Raises

This exercise will strengthen your shoulders and help you with routine lifting around the home. Start with your feet on the tubes and your hands by your side with your thumbs facing in toward your sides. Lift your arms up to the side straight out so you form a T. Your thumbs will be pointed downward as you get to the finishing position, so you'll feel resistance in your shoulders and stretching in your upper arm. Remember to bend your knees slightly.

Rowing

It's important to strengthen your back muscles to protect against back injury. This exercise will help you do that. Wrap the tube around a doorknob and then twist it so the tube is intertwined. You'll then want to slip the tube through the crack in the door as you close it. Squat slightly and with your palms down, begin a rowing motion, keeping your back straight and using mainly your arms and your back. There are tubes available, including the SPRI Xertube, that come with a door attachment. You can also wrap the tube around a bedpost or another immovable object.

Chest Press

Start by wrapping the tube around your back and make sure you have equal lengths in each hand. With your palms down, and your arms out to the side bent at 90 degrees at the elbow, push the handles forward in front of you. You'll feel the resistance in your chest and your pectoral muscles. You can work different parts of your pectoral muscles by moving the band up and down slightly on your back. And if you have a workout bench handy, you can try doing this exercise lying down to get even more resistance.

Remember with all of these exercises to drink plenty of fluids at room temperature before, during and afterward. Because there is only so much resistance you can get from the tubes, you might want to move on to other types of workouts. But before you do, make sure you've gotten the most out of these exercises.

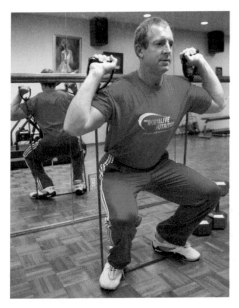

Squats

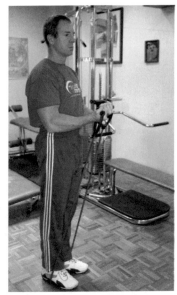

Curls

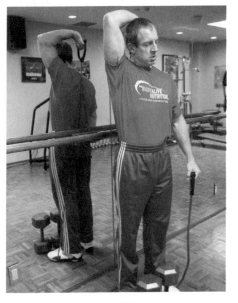

Tricep Press

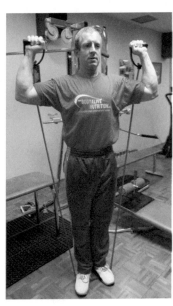

Lateral Raises

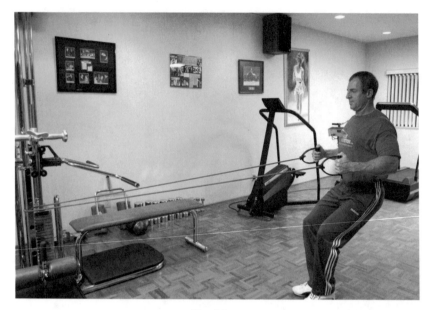

Rowing

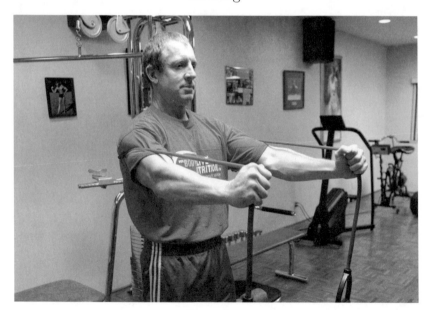

Chest Press

CHAPTER 24

THE SERETEAN ROUTINE

Going to the gym every day is something that works best for me, and I encourage others to make the trip if they can. Gyms can provide you with a broad selection of equipment, socialization and professional oversight you generally won't get anywhere else.

Most gyms, for example, have a wide variety of equipment you can use to exercise different muscle groups. In many cases, gyms offer several machines that exercise the same muscles, so you can choose the one that's best for you.

And gyms almost always have someone there who can keep an eye on you as you work out. There is also usually someone there to greet you as you walk in. While I tend to stay to myself when I'm working out, I do look forward to a brief chat with the gym staff every now and then.

One of the greatest advantages of going to a gym is that you have the ability to tap into the expertise of the staff. Most gyms have people available all of the time who are knowledgeable and well-trained on the equipment. The staffs are also available to help in an emergency situation, which is an important safety factor.

Gym membership fees vary, but in most cases you can find a facility in your area that is reasonably priced. Many offer discounts for seniors and sometimes significantly discounted memberships for daytime or off-peak times. You should be able to find memberships for less than $1 a day, which is a bargain if you go every day.

How often you go to the gym is up to you, but most personal trainers and physiologists will tell you that the more frequently you work out, the healthier you'll be. I make it a point to go to the gym every day and work out for a minimum of 50 minutes, but there are days when I don't make it because I'm traveling or not feeling well (rarely) or when I have family commitments. You shoot for 100 percent but accept 95 percent.

Before you begin working out at a gym, make sure you have the approval of your physician. And once you're at the gym, you should schedule an appointment with a personal trainer who can help you select the machines and starting weights that are right for you. A personal trainer will also teach you the proper technique to maximize your results and avoid injury. That's what I did and that's how the routine we're about to discuss was developed. Before we talk about the individual machines and exercises, there are a few things you should know.

I usually start my workout with aerobic exercises, including 12 to 13 minutes on the treadmill and 12 to 13 minutes on the stationary bike.

I then go to the machines and begin a weight-lifting cycle. I exercise on eight machines, doing 10 to 20 repetitions each. I move steadily from one machine to the next, making it into an aerobic effort as well as muscle building. Before the workout is over, I complete the cycle three times. By going through the cycle, rather than doing three sets on a machine at one time, you allow different sets of muscles to relax as you move from one machine to the other.

I also pay attention to my breathing. It's important that you exhale when you lift the weight to get the most benefit from the exercise. It's also important to make sure you lift the right amount of weight for you. Often it will be six months or more before I increase the weight on a certain machine. I make the change when the exercise becomes too easy and I can finish the 15 repetitions without difficulty. At the same time, if completing the 15 repetitions is too difficult, then you'll want to reduce the weights.

Here's my exercise routine:

Treadmill

I usually start on the treadmill, with my headset on, and adjust the speeds throughout the workout. I start at 3.8 miles per hour and peak at 4.2 miles an hour before decreasing my speed again. The schedule is as follows:

3.8 mph for 3 minutes
4 mph for 3 minutes
4.2 mph for 3 minutes
3.8 mph for 3 minutes

Stationary Bike

My goal is 25 minutes of aerobic exercise every day, so I usually work on the stationary bike for 12 to 13 minutes and strive to get my heart rate up to about 105, which is almost double my normal rate of 55. Once again, it's very important to consult professionals in helping you to determine a heart rate that is safe and optimal for you.

My pace on the stationary bike varies and is dictated by the music I'm listening to. I try to stay with the beat to keep a consistent pace. It's a fast pace since I listen to Latin salsa music. Three to four songs amount to 12 to 14 minutes. Listening to those songs instead of watching the clock helps take the boredom out of exercise. My headset, by the way, is a CD compressor. Currently I use the i-Pod. It stores 120 or so CDs, has great sound and weighs about 8 ounces.

Machine Exercises

The eight machines I use on a daily basis were selected for me by a personal trainer two years ago. When I have completed the circuit, I have exercised virtually all of my muscle groups.

I've been lifting weights for 10 years as a result of knowledge gained during a second visit to a Pritikin Center for a refresher course. The major differences from my first stay were the inclusion of weight lifting to the exercise regimen and a major improvement in the taste of the healthy food they serve.

Lateral Raise

The lateral raise is an exercise that has me pushing my elbows and using my deltoid muscles. I began this machine working with 60 pounds and I'm now up to 90 pounds.

Chest Press

I started this exercise – which works my pecs, deltoids and triceps – at 80 pounds and I'm now up to 120. In this exercise, I push forward to get resistance.

Rowing

Rowing is a great exercise in that it works several major muscle groups – back muscles, rhumboids, deltoids and shoulders – and also requires the use of other muscles, such as abdominal. On this machine, I'm now up to 120 pounds, having started at 90.

Shoulder Press

This is a simple exercise you do while sitting down. Lifting straight up with your arms slightly behind your head gives your shoulders a good workout. I'm up to 60 pounds now, having started at 40.

Arm Curls

This machine helps ensure you use the right form when doing arm curls that work the biceps. In doing this exercise, you'll give your abdominal muscles a workout as well. I started at 45 pounds and I'm now up to 60.

Pec Deck

This exercise works both the pectoral muscles and the deltoids and builds tone in the upper chest. I started with 40 pounds and am now at 60.

Seated Calf Raise

On this machine, I do 20 repetitions to build my calf and leg muscles. I'm up to 90 pounds after starting at 60.

Pull Downs

This is a great exercise for stretching your back and for working your arms and chest. Again, you also end up working your abdominal muscles. I started this with 80 pounds and I'm now up to 110.

Additional Exercise

In addition to my daily treadmill, bicycle exercises and weight-lifting routine, I walk the one-mile perimeter of my community three or four times a week. Four days of golf and practicing on the driving range complete my exercise regiment each week.

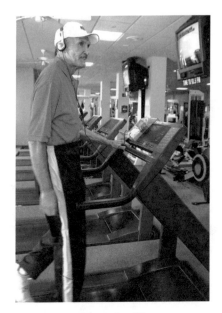

Treadmill

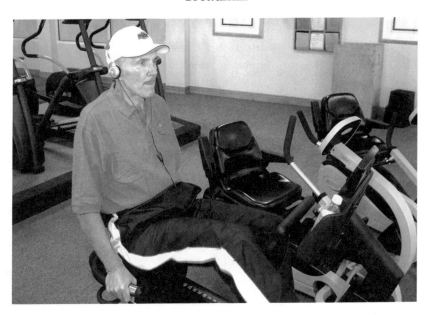

Stationary Bike

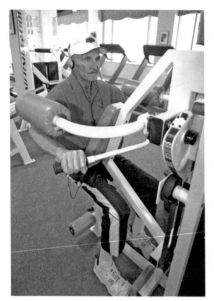

Lateral Raise

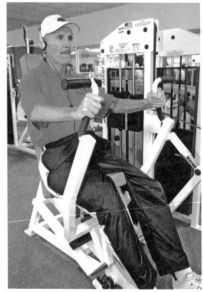

Chest Press

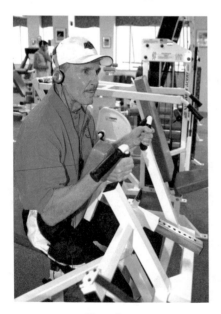

Rowing

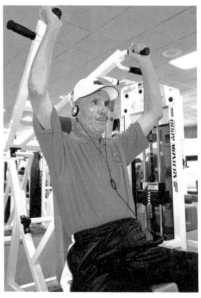

Shoulder Press

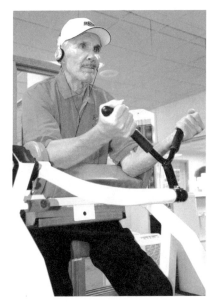

Arm Curls

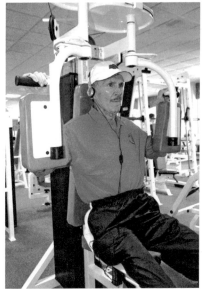

Pec Deck

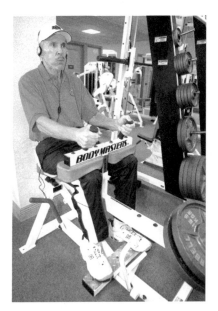

Seated Calf Raise

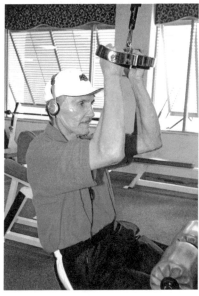

Pull Downs

CHAPTER 25

STAYING COMMITTED

As we all know, it's one thing to say we need to exercise but quite another to actually get started on a regular routine. And even when we do commit to exercise, staying motivated to stay physically fit for the rest of our lives can be just as challenging. As dedicated as I am to exercising 50 minutes a day, seven days a week, there are still some days when my motivation is a bit lacking. But over the years, I've discovered several ways to stay interested and true to my routine.

Perhaps my greatest motivation is the realization that by exercising I can add years to my life that will be good-quality years. There are studies upon studies, some of which we've already pointed out, showing that people who live a sedentary lifestyle are more prone to illness and disease. And while modern medicine makes it possible for us to live longer, it can't guarantee we'll live healthier. Exercise can't assure you'll live long either, but it's a big step in the right direction. The truth is, I'm certain I can have a better life 10 years down the road by spending 50 minutes a day exercising now. What better motivation is there than that?

One of the best things you can do to ensure you continue exercising is to get an exercise partner. If you're walking, set up a schedule so you and a partner, a spouse perhaps, walk on a regular basis. In many communities there are walking clubs and biking clubs, as well as swim clubs, where you have a regular schedule that encourages you to exercise with a group in a structured way. Aerobics classes or other exercise programs can also fill this need.

If you go to a gym, why not go with a friend if that will help you follow through on your commitment? While I do tend to work out by myself, I enjoy seeing the folks at my community fitness center on a regular basis and chatting briefly with them before beginning the workout.

For me, however, one of the best ways to stay motivated is to see the results of my efforts. That can mean maintaining my weight or achieving other goals I set for myself, such as reaching a certain Body Fat Index (BMI) or bringing my blood pressure down.

Of course, setting goals can be a double-edged sword. Your goals have to be realistic or you'll become frustrated and eventually stop exercising. A lot of people fail because they set their expectations too high. If you begin your workout and expect to lose 10 pounds in the first week, you'll be disappointed – and perhaps so discouraged that you might just give up. If you realize up front that it might take a month before you see any results, then you're more likely to stay with the program.

The concept that you'll lose weight immediately if you buy a certain machine or take a pill or exercise 20 minutes a day three days a week is crazy. The only way you'll lose weight is to burn more calories than you take in. If you set a target that's achievable and then achieve it, you'll get a sense of satisfaction that will serve as great motivation. Often people will use weight loss as a target, saying, for example, that they want to lose five pounds a month. But these are not the only goals you can work toward.

Goals I set for myself include:
- Lowering my cholesterol.
- Bringing down my pulse rate.
- Reducing my blood pressure.
- Lowering my BMI.
- Reducing my body fat.

I also find I can stay motivated by setting goals for each of the pieces of equipment I use in the gym. For example, I might decide I want to add 10 pounds to a particular weight-lifting machine within three or four weeks. I may also set a goal of building the number of miles I go on the exercise bike within a certain amount of time.

For many, it might be a good idea to talk to a personal trainer and find out what goals are realistic and achievable and also to make sure you're not overdoing it in an effort to reach a goal. A personal trainer can show you proper techniques that will help you get the most out of your exercise.

Once you've set your goals and gotten into your routine, you might need a little help fighting off boredom. There are some who enjoy listening to the radio or recorded music when they work out, others who read a book while on the treadmill, and still others who enjoy watching television.

Besides listening to music, I'll watch television, especially sporting events, while working out on the treadmill or bike because I can watch and still focus on what I'm doing. I'm not a big fan of listening to the radio while working out – too many distractions with commercials and music that might not be to my liking – nor do I like reading while on a bike or treadmill. But if it works for you, go ahead and do it.

Even with goals and entertainment, there might be days when you just don't feel like working out or doing your exercises. As with everything else, it's OK to take a vacation every now and then, but make sure it's not a long-term one. I give myself a guideline of taking off about 15 days a year, with the caveat that when I do feel good and have a bit more energy, I will add a little more to my exercise and try to make up for those lost days. And if you do skip the gym or the home workout, why not take a short walk, just to make sure you get some of the exercise you need?

While you're walking, or doing any other exercise, keep in mind how far you've come and the progress you've made. You'll feel good about what you've accomplished and that might be the best motivation of all.

CHAPTER 26

DOS AND DON'TS OF EXERCISE

- Don't overdo it. Don't do too much too fast. If you're doing weight training, start with lighter weights and reach a point where you feel strong resistance but not pain. When the workout is too easy and when you can easily do 15 repetitions, then increase resistance. If you can only make 10 repetitions, reduce the resistance.

- Don't work out on a full stomach. Wait at least 30 minutes after eating. After you eat, the digestive system demands an increased amount of oxygen and blood, which is diverted from your muscles. Straining those muscles during exercise, when they're deprived of the large amounts of oxygen needed, can be harmful.

- Do quickly inspect machines before using them. Make sure the weight is set properly before you use it if you work out at a gym or share your personal equipment. You should also check to make sure you're properly seated and check for frayed cables or anything else that could cause a problem.

- Do wear loose-fitting and well-ventilated clothing. Give your body a chance to sweat and lose heat through your pores during exercise. Wear clothing that allows for proper airflow but make sure it doesn't interfere with your workout.

- Do drink lots of room-temperature water. Drink water before, during and after your workout to make sure your muscles are properly hydrated. Drink water at room temperature because it's more easily absorbed than cold water.

DOS AND DON'TS OF EXERCISE

- Do be sure there's a phone within reach if you're exercising alone. That way you can summon help in the rare event of an emergency, especially if you're using a home gym or you're alone in a small workout room.

- Don't exercise after consuming alcohol. Alcohol tends to dehydrate your body, and of course, there's the possibility of impaired judgment. It just doesn't make sense to exercise after drinking.

- Don't exercise if you don't feel well. Give yourself a break. Exercising while ill can put additional pressure on a body that's already stressed.

- Do remember to stretch. Stretching your muscles before serious exercise can help you avoid cramping and muscle injuries. There are several different stretches you can do as outlined in an earlier chapter.

- Do warm up before resistance training. Eight to 10 minutes of cardiovascular exercise before you begin resistance training is important to prevent muscle soreness and injury.

PART III
WEIGHT

CHAPTER 27

MAINTAINING A HEALTHY WEIGHT

It happens to all of us.

At some point, usually in our 40s, we notice that the speed at which our bodies naturally burn calories – our metabolism – has slowed down. For some, that means going out and buying new pants with a little bigger waist size. For others it means a few more inches on the hips. As we get older and naturally more sedentary, we discover it's easy to add a few pounds here and there.

If there's any time to be keeping an eye on your weight, it should be as you move into and through your senior years. And remember, as I've said all along, it's never too late to start. Thumb through a book about people who have lived to be more than 100 years old and the chances are slim you'll find someone who's overweight. The truth is that the less weight you carry as you get older, the easier it is for your body to do its job.

There is, of course, an indisputable link between obesity and hypertension, diabetes and heart disease. The heavier you are, the harder your heart has to work to pump blood to the rest of your body. The heavier you are, the more pressure you put on your hips and knees, making it difficult for you to get around. That can begin a downward cycle to a more sedentary lifestyle.

The bottom line is this: the older we get, the more important it is to maintain a healthy weight. Not only will that help us feel better physically, but it will also help us look better, which of course can make us feel better. More importantly, maintaining a healthy weight will help us toward reaching our goal of living to 100 at a time when obesity is claiming more and more lives. Today obesity and excess weight are on the verge of bypassing cigarette smoking as the leading cause of preventable deaths in this country.

There are hundreds of gimmicks and gizmos out there designed to help you lose weight. There are probably more books on diets than on most other self-help topics, and there are more products out there promising to help you lose inches than you can imagine. There are the

171

supposedly magic pills, ultra weight-reducing milkshakes, and plans from self-proclaimed gurus who look like they haven't read their own books.

Now there's even stomach bypass surgery, endorsed by celebrities and TV weathermen. In my mind, the surgery is dangerous, expensive and unnecessary in 99 percent of the cases. There's no magic pill – no silver bullet – when it comes to losing weight and keeping it off. There's only one way to lose weight, and it requires some effort. You have to burn more calories than you take in.

It's a pretty simple concept. Things get a little more complicated when you try to figure out how to go about it. Most diets are just plans that help you reduce your calorie intake, either by eating less of certain types of foods or by eating less, period. But I don't believe diets alone will do the trick because they're generally just a temporary fix.

The type of food you eat must be combined with exercise to be effective over the long haul. It's as simple as that. If you only do half of the program, you'll be disappointed. As you know from reading all of the previous chapters, my focus is not on just diet or on just exercise, it's on the whole package. Living to 100 is not about diet fads or the latest fitness trends; it's about changing your attitude and living an overall healthy lifestyle.

Think about how much effort you'll waste if you spend several months on the South Beach Diet to shed 20 pounds and then go right back to eating the way you did before dieting. Remember, the best way to sustain positive weight loss is to change your lifestyle. Chances are if you transition to a healthy lifestyle from one that has been sedentary and filled with unhealthy food, your weight will come down automatically.

In this section I tell you about some of the most popular diets and share my thoughts on which ones might have merit. I also let you know which ones I think you should avoid and why. In the end, I hope this section provides insights you need to understand why it's important to maintain the weight that's right for you and how a healthy lifestyle will make that happen.

CHAPTER 28

MY WEIGHT STORY

By now, you've probably figured out I'm not a big proponent of diets to lose weight.

One reason is I don't think they really work. I would say that in 90 percent of the cases I'm familiar with, those who go on a diet end up gaining back whatever weight they lost within a matter of months. Then they try another diet or some pill promoted on a TV infomercial and another and another.

Our bodies were never meant to be treated in that fashion. I firmly believe it's important to keep an even keel – check the chart to find your ideal weight and stick with it. That target weight will eventually come down as we get older because it's normal to consume fewer calories as we age. If we continue on a regular exercise schedule, it makes weight loss easier.

There are ways to calculate our ideal weight, based on height and age, and ways to measure body fat. We'll talk about those later in this section. In most cases, we end up with a weight that is natural for us. Putting our bodies on a roller coaster of weight loss and gain, however, is not a natural way to maintain a healthy weight.

I'm very mindful of my weight, probably more than most people. I weigh myself on most mornings – always at the same time so comparisons are accurate. My target weight is 179 pounds, plus or minus three pounds. If I go over 182, I immediately cut back on my caloric intake for a day or two and I get back to my target weight. If I go under 176, I treat myself to a milkshake with skim milk and low-fat ice cream.

For me, my weight has never really been a problem, although there have been times in my life when I carried a few extra pounds. Back when I was in my 20s and going to college, I ate a lot of food and only exercised modestly. My weight shot up to 215 pounds. Still, the fact that I was 6-foot-4 hid my overweight condition.

During the last 26 years, since I started eating healthier and exercising regularly, I have tried to maintain a weight of 179 pounds. It's a weight that's best for my height and frame.

MY WEIGHT STORY

Maintaining a healthy weight isn't just about losing pounds. There are also times when it's important to build up your body. And gaining weight, in some circumstances, can be just as difficult and frustrating as losing it. Putting on pounds became a focus following surgery I underwent just before my 80th birthday. I lost 11 pounds in the hospital and knew I needed to gain it back as quickly as possible to maintain my strength. But because the body diverts a lot of its energy to healing following surgery or any other trauma, it's not always easy to get that weight back. Despite eating a lot more than usual, it took several months for me to return to my target weight.

Why is it so important to me to maintain the ideal weight? One reason is that I'm competitive and want to be as close to perfect as possible with all the numbers – cholesterol, weight, blood pressure. They are indicators of good health. By maintaining a target weight, we really do have a chance of reaching our goal of living to 100.

CHAPTER 29

THE IMPORTANCE
OF A HEALTHY WEIGHT

For decades, we have been told cigarette smoking resulted in the highest number of deaths in our nation. However, it's currently being challenged by the number of overweight-obesity-related deaths. In 2004, the U.S. Department of Health and Human Services estimated obesity and excess weight contributed to approximately 300,000 deaths a year, while cigarette smoking accounted for about 400,000. And the news keeps getting worse. Studies have shown the number of deaths related to obesity and excess weight continues to rise. Obesity is such a threat that the Surgeon General and other health officials made fighting it a top priority in 2001.

According to studies, the number of obese and overweight adults in the nation has more than doubled since 1980, to the point where nearly two-thirds of all adults are overweight. Obesity also has become a serious problem with children. The number of overweight children has tripled since 1980, and many school boards are reacting by offering healthier lunches and banning soda machines and snack machines from school grounds.

More importantly, at least for our purposes, is the fact that while obesity is also high among individuals over 55, our attitude may be a little more lackadaisical than that of other age groups. We need to be more vigilant about maintaining a healthy weight if we want to continue living a healthy and active life.

A 2003 study of 1,100 adults over age 65 found that more than half could be considered overweight or obese. Yet most of the people in the study said they were happy or very happy with their weight. In the study, 20 percent of those who were overweight actually thought they were underweight or normal, while 46 percent of those who were overweight said they were satisfied with their weight. In the group surveyed, a little more than half said they were less worried about gaining weight now than they had been in the past.

THE IMPORTANCE
OF A HEALTHY WEIGHT

One of the findings that concerned me was a conclusion that seniors who are overweight are more likely than those who are not overweight to try to shed pounds by eating more protein or by skipping meals. In my mind, neither of those alternatives should even be considered because they don't work and they're not as good for your health as a long-term change to a healthy lifestyle.

The results of the study come as no surprise. Day in and day out, I hear from friends and family members that at their age it is too late to worry about being too heavy. They are, in essence, giving up and saying that since they're in their 70s and don't have much time left, they aren't going to worry about being overweight.

Even our doctors are sometimes lax in their efforts to help us change our lifestyles. Too often physicians will say that because we are of a certain age, in our twilight years, we need not worry about losing those extra pounds. Also, sad to say, many doctors are overweight themselves, making it awkward for them to recommend weight-reduction programs.

But there are a lot of good reasons to worry, especially if you want to make it to your 80s and beyond. As I've mentioned before, it is never too late to start reversing the harmful effects of an unhealthy lifestyle. Losing weight in your 60s, 70s or 80s will help extend your life.

By now you must know being overweight or obese is associated with everything from heart disease and cancer to bad joints. Studies have shown that people who are obese have a 50 percent to 100 percent greater chance of dying earlier from all causes than those who are not. The study shows that seniors who are obese can shave anywhere from two to five years off their lives, while those in their 20s who are obese could shorten their lives by nine to 13 years.

According to studies from the National Institutes of Health, obesity and excess weight are known risks for diabetes, heart disease, stroke, hypertension, gallbladder disease, osteoarthritis, sleep apnea and some forms of cancer.

Here are some interesting statistics from a variety of studies highlighted by the NIH:

- Among those who have Type 2 diabetes, almost 70 percent are overweight and almost 50 percent are obese.

THE IMPORTANCE
OF A HEALTHY WEIGHT

- About 27 percent of all overweight adult men and 32 percent of overweight women suffer from high blood pressure, compared with 15 percent for both men and women who are not overweight. Those who are obese have a greater chance of suffering from high blood pressure, with 42 percent of obese men and 38 percent of obese women being diagnosed as hypertensive.

- While about 13 percent of adults who are not overweight suffer from high cholesterol, the percentage of obese men with high cholesterol is about 22 percent, while that number climbs to 27 percent in obese women.

- Although there is still much work to be done on the link between cancer and obesity, one study concluded that cancer death rates were 52 percent higher in obese men than in those who were not considered overweight and 62 percent higher in obese women. The study also showed a higher death rate from certain types of cancer, including colon and esophagus cancer, in those who were obese.

Physicians will also tell you being overweight can mean you're at a greater risk should you require surgery.

Once again, the facts confirm just how important it is to maintain a healthy weight and how detrimental being overweight or obese can be to your overall well being. But it's never too late to set about reversing the damage and moving toward a healthier lifestyle with exercise and proper nutrition.

CHAPTER 30

THE PROS AND CONS
OF VARIOUS DIETS

The focus in this book is on living a healthy lifestyle. That's why the Nutrition section recommends a lifelong way of eating healthy rather than any particular short-term diet. It is one of the keys to staying healthy while living longer.

Many people have lost weight dieting. But often it's only a temporary fix to an ongoing problem because foremost in so many dieters' minds is the idea that once you reach the desired weight, you can stop dieting – which is why so often people eventually gain back what they lose. In fact, they often gain more than they lost because dieting tends to slow down metabolism, so it's more difficult to lose on each succeeding diet. This yo-yo, up-and-down pattern can injure your health over time.

At any given time, someone you know will probably be on a diet – at least that's been my experience. The diet business generates about $33 billion in sales annually in the United States, according to the American Dietetic Association. Walk into any bookstore, supermarket or drugstore and you'll find a proliferation of diet books, cookbooks, nutritional supplement books and similar products.

So here's a quick rundown on a few of the most popular diets, and my perspective on them.

Weight Watchers

The current Weight Watchers diet plans are based on either a points system called the Flex Plan or the Core Plan, which focuses on eating from a core group of certain healthy foods. Under the points system, various foods have been given a point value according to type and portion size. The more calories, the more points. Fat adds to the points, while fiber subtracts from them. The core system limits what foods people can eat but allows them to avoid having to track food intake.

This diet program has been around for a long time and a lot of people have lost weight on it and kept it off. While today it's possible to

178

join online, a key to Weight Watchers' success has been the way it has traditionally worked. People gather once a week in a class setting, get weighed, receive advice from the class leader and discuss how they're doing on the diet. This system helps provide support and encouragement for people to achieve their weight-loss goals.

The point system makes it simple for dieters to keep track of what they're eating. While there's no restriction on the type of food they can eat, they are encouraged to eat healthily and to take advantage of low-sugar or artificially sweetened desserts, and of low- or non-fat products, which have a lower point value than, for example, whole milk.

Early in the plan, the dieters receive a booklet about how to exercise and what levels of activity are considered low, moderate or vigorous. Dieters can gain additional daily points based on their level and frequency of exercise.

The core diet eliminates such foods as fruit and vegetable juices, cream soups, french fries and fruit packed in syrup. Core foods include fruits and vegetables without added sugar, fat or sauce, as well as whole grains, unrefined cereals and lean meats, but limits them to one serving a day.

There's an emphasis on eating healthy foods and including essential oils in the eating plans, although they do not specifically address omega 3 oils. Eating non-fat and sugar-free foods is encouraged although not required on the points plan. The core plan, however, requires most of these foods.

Dr. Phil McGraw's Ultimate Weight Solution

Phillip C. McGraw, Ph.D., is a psychologist who became a celebrity after frequent appearances on the Oprah Winfrey talk show, which ultimately led him to his own television show. Published in 2003, *The Ultimate Weight Solution* was his first book on weight loss.

Dr. Phil, as he is popularly called, is known for his straightforward, sometimes tough, no-nonsense advice on life and its problems. In fact, the first two chapters of his weight-loss book are called "Getting Real About You and Your Weight" and "Get-Real Expectations and Goals."

His approach is not too scientific. He sees eating basically as behavioral; consequently, *The Ultimate Weight Solution* is written a lot like a self-help book. Dr. Phil provides little quizzes along the way to assess what the dieter needs to focus on and urges a positive mental approach toward losing weight. He outlines seven " keys" to permanent weight loss. Among these are Right Thinking, Healing Feelings, A No-fail Environment, and Intentional Exercise. He says he's telling people how to program their lives to achieve their weight-loss goals.

The book has a variety of plans to confront problems the dieter may encounter and advises readers what to expect when embarking on a new diet. Dr. Phil divides food into either high-yield (healthy) or low-yield (unhealthy) status and lists those that fall into these categories. He suggests eliminating unhealthy foods by not having them in the house, and provides a series of suggested meal plans but no recipes. However, he really isn't too specific on why you should or shouldn't eat certain foods.

I can't help thinking Dr. Phil's diet doesn't go far enough. For instance, while he advises against eating unhealthy fats, he also says not to put too much butter or margarine on rolls. But why suggest any food that has bad stuff such as saturated fat or trans fat even on a limited basis? Why include them in a diet at all?

The Atkins Diet

In 1972, the late Dr. Robert C. Atkins published *Dr. Atkins' Diet Revolution – The High Calorie Way to Stay Thin Forever*, which suggested a radical approach to losing weight. Atkins, a New York cardiologist, claimed the best and healthiest way to lose weight and keep it off was to be on a high-fat, high-protein and low-carbohydrate diet. He revised the book in 1992 as *Dr. Atkins' New Diet Revolution*, which set off the current low-carbohydrate craze and also precipitated a barrage of other "low-carb" diets, diet books and cookbooks.

The Atkins diet has four phases, beginning with the induction phase, where dieters are encouraged to eat all the fat, dairy and protein they want but little else other than about a half-cup of salad daily. This is supposed to bring about ketosis, a state in which the body begins to burn fat for energy instead of glucose. Over the next three phases, more carbohydrates are introduced, including some grains, many more vegetables and some fruits.

The diet seems to work for some people, who have lost weight and, if they adhere to the maintenance plan for the diet, do keep it off. However, studies have shown that while people may experience rapid weight loss at the beginning of this diet, over a year's period of time there's only about the same amount of weight loss as there is on other diets such as Weight Watchers.

Atkins was aware early on of the dangers of refined carbohydrates and included talks about them even in his 1972 book. His philosophy was that refined carbohydrates are a major contributor to excessive weight, obesity, coronary heart disease, diabetes and various other serious health problems. I couldn't agree more.

What I don't agree with, however, is his argument that all carbohydrates contribute to this problem, although perhaps to a lesser degree. It's my belief, backed by most of the scientific community, that the majority of unrefined and/or complex carbohydrates, including whole grains, vegetables and fruits, are good for you and contribute to good health. Atkins recommended nutritional supplements to replace some missing nutrients. But what other important ones are we missing when we significantly limit our intake of foods with healthy carbohydrates, such as vegetables?

Nor do I believe it's OK to eat unlimited amounts of steak, cream, butter, regular cheese and so forth, encouraged on the Atkins regimen. I believe – again in keeping with most current scientific thought – that, with the exception of some healthy monounsaturated and polyunsaturated fats such as omega-3s, we should be keeping our intake of fats to a minimum, especially saturated fats and trans fats.

In addition, diets high in saturated fats and trans fats are well known in the medical field to lead to clogged arteries, a significant factor in the development of heart disease and stroke.

Another serious problem to me is the lack of significant, long-term, studies done on the Atkins diet. There's an ongoing debate in the medical community about the long-term effects of the diet in regard to kidney function, cholesterol levels, and the potential for an increased risk of osteoporosis, heart disease and cancer.

The South Beach Diet

The South Beach Diet was written by Dr. Arthur Agatston, a Miami Beach cardiologist who had been prescribing it for his patients for a number of years before he wrote the book. It has two main phases. The first, which usually lasts about two weeks, resembles the induction phase of the Atkins Diet in that it prohibits bread, rice, sugars or pasta. However, it does allow vegetables, such as salads and green beans, along with lean meats, chicken and fish (grilled or broiled), nuts and eggs.

Later, whole grains, additional vegetables and some fruits are added. While the South Beach Diet is sometimes described as a low-carb and low-fat diet, it actually tends to focus away from unhealthy fats and refined, processed and fried foods. It also recommends mostly complex carbohydrates, and includes vegetables, some fruits and low-fat protein products.

It doesn't focus on counting carbohydrates but mainly on the Glycemic Index, that is, to what degree a food raises blood sugar – because generally, current scientific thought suggests that the faster blood sugar is raised, the hungrier people can get, which may lead to overeating. It allows seafood, chicken breast, lean meat, low-fat cheese, most vegetables, nuts, oils, whole grains, most fruits, low-fat milk and yogurt, and beans. It limits fatty meats, regular cheese, refined grains, juice, potatoes and sweets.

CHAPTER 31

DETERMINING YOUR IDEAL BODY WEIGHT

Are you overweight? You might not think so, but you could be wrong. Studies have shown a large percentage of those who are overweight according to generally accepted standards don't believe they are.

So how do you know? For years, physicians and insurance companies would calculate your ideal weight based on your height. One of the old standards was the Metropolitan Life Insurance Company chart that's still in use today.

Desirable Weights For Men Over 25				*Desirable Weights For Women Over 25*			
Height	**Frame**			**Height**	**Frame**		
	Small	Medium	Large		Small	Medium	Large
5' 2"	112-120	118-129	126-141	4' 10"	92-98	96-107	104-119
5' 3"	115-123	121-133	129-141	4' 11"	94-101	98-110	105-122
5' 4"	118-126	124-138	132-148	5' 0"	96-104	101-103	109-125
5' 5"	121-129	127-139	135-152	5' 1"	99-107	104-118	112-128
5' 6"	124-133	134-147	142-161	5' 2"	102-110	107-119	115-131
5' 7"	128-137	134-147	142-161	5' 3"	105-113	110-127	118-134
5' 8"	132-141	138-152	147-168	5' 4"	108-118	113-126	121-138
5' 9"	138-145	142-158	151-170	5' 5"	111-119	116-130	125-142
5' 10"	140-150	146-180	155-174	5' 6"	114-123	120-135	129-146
5' 11"	144-154	150-165	159-179	5' 7"	118-127	124-139	133-150
6' 0"	148-158	154-170	164-184	5' 8"	122-131	128-143	137-154
6' 1"	152-162	158-175	168-189	5' 9"	126-135	132-147	141-158
6' 2"	156-167	162-180	173-194	5' 10"	130-140	138-151	145-163
6' 3"	160-171	167-185	178-199	5' 11"	134-144	140-155	149-168
6' 4"	164-175	172-190	182-204	6' 1"	138-148	144-159	153-173

Now, however, the USDA Dietary Guide for Americans uses the Body Mass Index (BMI) standard to determine ideal weight. You can calculate your BMI by plugging your height and weight into a mathematical equation, or by looking at the following chart.

DETERMINING YOUR
IDEAL BODY WEIGHT

Here's how you do it. Divide your weight in pounds by your height in inches. Divide that number by your height in inches and then multiply that number by 703.

ARE YOU AT A HEALTHY WEIGHT?

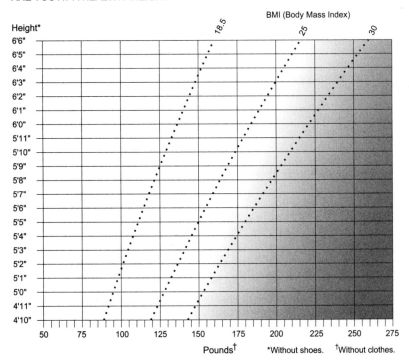

BMI (Body Mass Index)

Pounds†   *Without shoes.   †Without clothes.

To set health guidelines using BMI, researchers looked at mortality information and concluded that those with a BMI above 25 are at a higher risk of earlier death than those with a BMI below 25.

The consensus among most in the nutrition community is that those with a BMI between 25 and 30 are overweight and those with a BMI above 30 are obese.

But it's not that simple, at least in my mind. For instance, whether you're calculating BMI or healthy weight based just on height, you need to take into consideration the size of your frame.

DETERMINING YOUR
IDEAL BODY WEIGHT

A person who is 6-foot-3 with a narrow frame like mine, for example, should weigh less than someone the same height and built like a football player. While the Metropolitan chart takes that into consideration, the BMI doesn't. Nor does the BMI take gender into consideration, something the Metropolitan chart does.

And, then of course, there's the importance of factoring in your age. It's my belief that as we age we should actually weigh less than the charts show. That way, our heart, joints and other organs won't have to work as hard to keep us functioning on a daily basis. Just about all the centenarians I have met or read about over the years are small and thin. Comedian George Burns comes to mind.

But there are other things to consider in determining your ideal weight. Two important factors are how you really feel and how concerned you are about your appearance. If you like to look trim, you might want to go below your ideal weight and stay there. Then again, you can stray from your ideal weight by plus or minus three to five pounds at any given time and not be concerned.

I do think it's important to find the weight that's right for you and be vigilant about maintaining it. I would suggest you check your weight once a week and keep a record of it.

CHAPTER 32
STAYING WITH IT

You know you have to lose weight and keep it off. You even know the target weight you need to reach and maintain. Now all you have to do is make up your mind you're going to get into a healthy lifestyle program and stay with it, with a major goal of getting to and maintaining your recommended weight.

Maintaining a healthy weight is one of the biggest challenges most people face because your weight loss comes easier at first than it does later on. In the long run, however, it's the rewards you don't see right away – the probability of staving off heart disease, diabetes, cancer and joint deterioration – that may have the greatest impact on the length and quality of your life.

So how do you go about keeping off the weight you dropped during a healthy weight-loss regimen? Once again, there's no magic pill. Scientists are forever working to find one, but I wouldn't hold my breath. If there were, the great majority of dieters who experience the yo-yo effect of weight loss wouldn't be going through all those ups and downs. I've seen different people use various techniques to keep the weight they've lost from coming back. In general, those who have the most success keeping weight off have done so by making a commitment and maintaining the habits they picked up while living a healthier lifestyle.

In a 2004 series of articles on obesity, *Time* magazine reported on studies of more than 5,000 people who made it onto the National Weight Control Registry by losing more than 30 pounds and keeping it off for longer than one year. While the studies showed that those who were successful used different techniques to shed their pounds – some going cold turkey, others using organized programs – there were several common denominators that helped them keep the weight off. Most of those on the registry made it a point to add physical exercise to their lifestyle in order to lose weight, in addition to reducing their calorie intake and possibly reducing the fat in their diet. Walking was by far the exercise of choice, but many decided to take up other physical activities as well, including swimming, hiking and biking.

Once they reached their target weight, those with the most success at losing weight continued to stay with the physical exercise. The runners kept running and the walkers kept walking. They also continued to monitor their calorie intake and kept a vigilant eye on their weight, most checking the scale every week.

Most of those on the registry made it a point to eat breakfast every day, a factor experts say helps you lose weight because it lowers your chance of eating unhealthy snacks. I've also noticed many people who lose weight continue to eat smaller portions once they reach their goal in order to keep the weight off.

What struck me, after reading the *Time* article, is that the people most successful at losing weight were those who were the most motivated to do so. To them, keeping the weight off became an important focus in their lives. It's much like what we've been talking about all through these chapters.

If living healthy becomes part of your everyday lifestyle, then keeping the weight off will come naturally. For me, weight has never really been an issue, but I'm competitive and I enjoy the challenge of setting a goal and staying with it. I like looking at the scale every week and knowing I've achieved my goal of keeping my weight where I want it to be. For some, reaching a weight goal also helps you feel better about the way you look.

My guess is those who make it to the national registry of weight losers are proud of what they've achieved and don't want to see all of their achievements disappear. We look at how far we've come and we realize how easy it is to stay there just by doing the things we've already come to enjoy. Knowing what we know about the effects of excess weight and the impact it has on our overall health, I can't understand why more of us over the age of 55 aren't working harder to keep the pounds down.

After all, we can live longer, enjoy life to its fullest and set a healthy example for our families. In many ways, maintaining a healthy weight is just as important as shaking the smoking habit.

CHAPTER 33

THE COST OF BEING
OVERWEIGHT OR OBESE

A few years ago, studies were done to determine how much obesity costs the country in terms of actual direct costs, such as health-care charges, and indirect costs, such as lost wages. The National Institutes of Health adjusted the costs into current dollars in 2001 and these figures continue to grow. It's estimated that between $75 billion and $90 billion each year is spent on the direct medical costs for treating those who have medical conditions related to excess weight. As I mentioned, that can be anything from having knees and hips replaced to diabetes and heart disease.

On top of that, there's another $12 billion in indirect costs to private employers, so the estimated costs of obesity and excess weight can exceed $100 billion each year. Those indirect costs include lower productivity of employees, increased absenteeism and increases in health insurance premiums. According to studies, work time lost due to obesity costs employers an estimated $40 million a year, while doctor visits related to excess weight cost employers an estimated $63 million each year. Companies lose an estimated $239 million each year because employees who are overweight can't perform all of their expected job duties.

While I have not found any studies that directly link the amount of money Medicare spends each year as a result of obesity and excess weight, my guess is that the number is significant since Medicare and Medicaid pay for 23 percent of the nation's health-care bill. The impact of that, of course, is an escalation of the depletion of Medicare funds and eventually an increase to the taxpayers.

Taxpayers also end up paying more into state Medicaid funds due to excess weight, as those funds are designed to assist people who are financially struggling. Since research shows those living in poverty have a higher-than-average rate of obesity, it's probably safe to conclude Medicaid would pay a lot less if we were able to eliminate problems related to obesity and excess weight.

THE COST OF BEING
OVERWEIGHT OR OBESE

If that news isn't startling enough, here's a prediction that should concern everyone. Researchers believe unless something is done to control the obesity epidemic, the proportion of health-care dollars spent on excess weight-related illnesses will increase more than 20 percent by 2010. The bottom line is that all of us, even those who never have a weight problem, end up paying for those who suffer illnesses related to excess weight.

According to studies cited by the National Institutes of Health, the greatest amount of money spent on illnesses related to excess weight is on treating those with Type 2 diabetes. Next in line is heart disease. Studies show about 17 percent of the total amount of money spent each year treating heart disease, or about $8.8 billion, is related to excess weight.

Think about how many bypass surgeries and angioplasty treatments we could avoid if we were able to reduce obesity in this country. The amount of money saved would be huge. Studies also show the total costs, direct and indirect, of excess weight among those who suffer from osteoarthritis are estimated to be about $21 billion a year. The bulk of that amount, about 75 percent, is because of lost productivity, absenteeism and increased insurance premiums.

The cost of treating those with cancer who are overweight is more than $2 billion and the indirect costs of cancer, related to excess weight are more than $3 billion. At this point, we should probably talk about the intangible costs of these diseases. Look at the impact these diseases have on those who are suffering from them and their loved ones. When you look at the total costs of excess weight, it doesn't take a genius to figure out that everyone, especially those of us over 55 who have knowledge and time, should do something about it. And now is the time to start.

Before I close this chapter, I want to share another number with you. Each year, according to some studies, Americans spend an estimated $33 billion on weight-loss products. That number represents how much we spend on diet foods and commercial diet programs, not to mention diet books and other weight-loss-related products. Wouldn't it be better if that money was spent on a healthier lifestyle that includes more exercise and healthier food?

CHAPTER 34

DOS AND DON'TS FOR MAINTAINING A HEALTHY WEIGHT

- Don't get taken in by fad diets that include high-fat or other unhealthy foods.

- Don't go on a fad diet and expect to lose weight and keep it off without exercise.

- Don't forget obesity is linked to many diseases that can be fatal.

- Do remember the older we get, the more important it is to maintain a healthy weight.

- Don't get caught in a cycle of losing weight, gaining it back and then losing it again.

- Do remember the only real way to lose weight is to burn more calories than you take in.

- Do determine the weight that's best for you based on your height, frame and gender or on your Body Mass Index.

- Don't worry about being two or three pounds over or under your ideal healthy weight if you're getting adequate exercise.

- Do remember weight-loss diets might help you shed a few pounds, but reverting to a healthy lifestyle can keep you fit.

- Do remember weight-loss quick fixes and miraculous "silver bullets" are more likely to shrink your wallet than your waistline and do little to help you live a healthy lifestyle.

PART IV
STRESS

CHAPTER 35

MANAGING YOUR STRESS

The question was asked innocently.

How could retirees – people who should be enjoying a life of leisure, the perfect life – possibly get stressed out?

The truth is there's a lot to be stressed about as you get older. Sure, you might not have job-related stress or the problems that come from raising children, but there could be family problems and sickness and, for some, financial issues that can be overwhelming. As we get older, the stresses change but they still exist.

For some, caring for an ailing spouse can be tremendously stressful and for others it's easy to become stressed about how the children are doing. Unfortunately, there are people whose lives are cut short because they're actually stressed about dying. Ironically, concerns about your health can lead you to become more stressed. And becoming more stressed will likely take its toll on your health.

Researchers believe stress can accelerate the aging of the brain and can in fact lead to an impairment of the cognitive functions. And of course, stress can lead to aging in other parts of the body as well. It's believed stress leads to the release of free radicals, which contribute to cell damage. There is also the impact of adrenaline, a stimulant to the nervous system, running through your body in reaction to what's called the "fight or flight response." Doctors and cardiologists know stress is a key risk factor in heart disease. Researchers believe people who are angry or chronically stressed are more likely to suffer a heart attack or become victims of cancer.

Of all the risk factors for heart disease, stress might be the one most of us would be motivated enough to control.

Stress is something all of us go through. Some people, however, handle it better than others. Stress is something you can't avoid, but you can control it.

In this section of the book, I'll talk about stress and about things you might want to consider to better manage it. We've already discussed how exercise can ease stress, and in this section we'll talk a little about things like imagery and visualization. We'll also discuss some deep-breathing techniques that are useful. We'll even talk about how pets can help you feel more relaxed.

But to really control stress, to really learn how to manage it, you have to have the right attitude. Perhaps that attitude is best summed up in two ways. The first is in a quote that was attributed to Art Linkletter, who said: "Things turn out best for those who make the best out of the way things turn out." His point is that if you accept things the way they are and make the best of them, you'll be less stressed and probably live a little longer.

The next bit of advice comes from the Serenity Prayer. You might recall that the prayer asks for "...serenity to accept the things I cannot change; courage to change the things I can; and wisdom to know the difference."

The truth is that, as the prayer says, if there's something you can do nothing about, you have to learn how to ensure it doesn't cause you stress. I believe if you can develop this technique, you can eliminate half the stress in your life.

But even if you can't, that doesn't mean you are without alternatives.

Throughout my life, I've found myself in many stressful situations, both personal and professional.

In my professional life, I made it a point to get to know virtually all of the employees of Coronet, the carpet company I headed. When I had to lay off people because of a slowdown in the economy, it was the worst feeling in the world. I didn't cope well with the stress. These were not only my employees who'd helped me build the business, but they were my friends. I slept only three or four hours a night with a pad of paper next to the bed so I could make notes on business decisions or personal problems. I often suffered stomach pains from overeating junk food. The pains became so severe, I often doubled over in the office and had to lie down on a couch to get relief.

It was about that time I realized another key rule in managing stress: if a situation is too stressful, avoid it whenever possible. Of course you can't always avoid stressful situations. Getting stuck in traffic is something you generally can't plan on. But if you know you don't handle the stress of traffic well, then make plans to take roads that will be less congested. You might lose minutes on your trip, but you could add years onto your life.

MANAGING YOUR STRESS

Knowing yourself is critical to reducing your stress level. Think about it for a few minutes and assess the things in life that create negative stress for you. Then think of ways to avoid them. And remember there are always situations where you can just walk away if you feel yourself getting riled up.

These days, I'm much less likely to become stressed than I was 10 or 15 years ago. There are a number of reasons. For one thing, I'm motivated to manage my stress effectively. Years ago, I wasn't really aware, or perhaps didn't really care, that stress was bad for my health. Today, I realize how bad stress is for my health and I know if I want to live to 100 and beyond, I'd better manage it. In this section, we'll talk about ways to look at stress and steps you can take to reduce it.

CHAPTER 36

MY STORY ABOUT MANAGING STRESS

All of us have stress. It's a fact. The truth is no matter who you are – whether you're the head of a major corporation or a retiree driving an RV across the country – chances are sooner or later you'll face an unexpected situation that will cause you some anxiety. How we manage that stress depends on who we are and perhaps on how much we concern ourselves with keeping stress to a minimum.

Over the years, many books and educational courses have been developed on stress management. I've discovered there's no easy approach that works for everyone. If there were, we'd certainly be a less-stressful nation. Instead, each of us has to find ways to manage our own stress – ways that work best for us.

Throughout this section, you'll find information that might help you learn to manage your stress. And while I can't offer you a guaranteed way to relieve anxiety, I can tell you about the stresses in my life and how I've come to deal with them. During my stays at a Pritikin Longevity Center and later while attending programs run by Dr. Dean Ornish, I became very aware stress was bad for my health. Now I know stress is a silent killer, especially for someone like me, once classified as a hyper, Type-A personality.

Staying healthy is a very important part of my life, and I know in order to do that I have to be especially mindful to avoid stress. In many ways, stress is just like eating a burger with fries. It's one more thing that's bad for me and should be avoided. Knowing that, and really believing it, helps keep me motivated to manage my own stress. Up until the time I went to the Pritikin Longevity Center, I don't think I realized or really cared about the ill effects stress was having on my body.

As a youngster, I had the typical youthful stresses, such as schoolwork, getting a date, and in my case, getting rid of acne. Stress at that time in my life didn't result in any physical damage.

While I was in the Army during World War II, I don't think I understood the full impact of the stress that came from not knowing where

MY STORY ABOUT MANAGING STRESS

I was going to be stationed or what I'd be doing next. The uncertainty that filled my years in the military from 1942 to 1946 brought all kinds of stress. There was a sense that we had no control of our lives. On the other hand, I was with thousands of other guys and because we were all in the same boat, sometimes literally, we could often kid about our situation, which sometimes eased the stress.

After coming back from the military, I went to college and discovered a whole new set of stresses. I had to make up time since I'd lost four years due to my military service, and I had a lot of ground to cover. I focused my efforts on getting good grades because I knew I wanted to go to graduate school. The stress of having to compete for good grades stayed with me even after I got into New York University and worked towards a master's degree.

One of the most stressful times in my life came as I was preparing to leave graduate school and move into the real world. Because I had excellent grades at NYU and excellent grades at Oklahoma State, both of which complemented a reasonably impressive resume, I figured I'd have no problem getting a good job. I just assumed it would be a question of which job offer I'd accept. I interviewed at the top three department stores in New York, and even though they accepted a total of 15 students from my class, I was not hired. I was embarrassed and devastated but made up my mind I would make each one of those businesses regret not hiring me.

Over time I accomplished that goal, but it took a lot of hard work accompanied by a lot of stress. Throughout those days, and during the years when I was building a business by investing everything I owned into it, the stress factor was constant and growing.

Well, how did I get through these stressful periods in my life? One tool was humor. Laughter is always a great weapon in the arsenal of stress reducers. Throughout most of my life, I've always looked for the lighter side of things and enjoyed sharing a laugh with family or friends.

Laughter, as you may be aware, is also a great tool in protecting your health. Studies have shown that laughter can have a positive impact on reversing some illnesses.

A recent study at the University College London of 227 men and women found that people who were happier had healthier levels of stress hormones and, as a result, were less likely to suffer from heart disease as well as inflammatory ailments.

MY STORY ABOUT MANAGING STRESS

Your attitude, I've discovered, is critical to your health. Over the years I've learned that taking a positive approach can help minimize stress.

I've also learned the value of walking away. When I was running my company, I had a very wise assistant who kept me out of trouble. There would be times when I'd get all riled up and dictate a letter full of fire and probably a lot of things I didn't really want to say. Overnight I'd think about the letter and realize my words would probably do more harm than good. I would fret about the impact the letter would have on a business relationship. Invariably, when I'd get to the office I'd discover that my assistant had an excuse for why she hadn't been able to get the letter out the day before. The original letter would end up in the trash, replaced by a more effective one reflecting a more conciliatory tone.

Another lesson I've learned is that it's stressful to react immediately during a stressful situation. So whenever possible, I now make it a point to walk away from these kinds of situations. I don't avoid them completely. Instead, I try to get busy with something else and then pick up the next morning where I left off.

As I mentioned earlier, there were some stressful times when I was running the company and I learned the best way to handle stress can often be to redirect your energies into less-stressful activities.

After the company was acquired by RCA Corp., I opted to pursue a career in professional sports, where I thought I'd have more fun and less stress. I became president and general manager of the Atlanta Hawks basketball team. After we lost a game, I'd replay that game overnight in my head four or five times, thinking about how we could have done things better. The wins were fun but the losses were more stressful than what I had experienced in running a company. After two years, I decided it would be better to just attend the games and let someone else run the team.

During times when I find myself wound up or having trouble sleeping, I rely on a few tried-and-true techniques to help me relax.

The first, and the easiest for most people, is deep breathing. Sometimes when I'm lying in bed trying to fall asleep or trying to relax, I start doing deep-breathing exercises. With my mouth open, I inhale slowly, counting to eight before I stop. I hold my breath for eight counts and then exhale, counting to 16. I repeat this several times until I feel relaxed.

One of the additional benefits of deep breathing is it helps get more oxygen to your brain. As a result, you're usually able to think a bit more clearly. Many researchers believe deep breathing is extremely effective in stressful situations because it helps you make better decisions.

The second technique I use is called imagery. It's an extremely effective technique taught at the Pritikin Longevity Center. Here's how it works: as I'm lying in bed, I think about the blood that's going through my body. Then starting at my head, I imagine the blood draining from my muscles, causing them to relax and go limp. I do this one muscle group at a time and work my way down to my toes. Using this technique, I can actually lower my pulse rate as well as my blood pressure.

Another technique is visualization. I recapture stress-free moments of my life, thereby distracting me from what caused me to feel stressed in the first place. For example, when I was vacationing in the Bahamas, I remember lying in a hammock on a partially deserted beach listening to the waves, seeing the palm trees sway in the wind and falling asleep.

I keep that occasion in my mind, and by putting myself back in that hammock from time to time, I can relieve my stress.

Another technique I've found useful is muscle relaxation. I tense each muscle as tightly as I can, then release it and let it go limp. I do this one muscle group at a time, starting with my toes.

These techniques seem to work for me. They may work for you. The important thing is to find the best techniques to help you manage your own stress.

CHAPTER 37

STRESS - WHAT IS IT?

When most of us think of stress, we tend to think of it in negative terms. But stress can also be positive. Understanding the difference between positive and negative stress, and knowing how to get more out of positive stress while reducing its negative counterpart, can be important to long-term health.

So what is stress? In simple terms, it's the body's reaction to a perceived threat – not necessarily a real threat. As our bodies evolved, we developed mechanisms to protect us from dangers ranging from a charging beast to a toxic microscopic virus.

In essence, our brain, once alerted to a danger, sends out signals that prepare almost every part of our body to ward off or minimize the impact of the attack. When we're stressed, increased amounts of adrenaline flow through the body, leading to an increased heart rate. Meanwhile, other chemicals are released that do everything from making our blood stickier so a wound will clot faster to increasing fat cells in case we're not able to reach our food supply. All of this takes place in an instant.

Some researchers believe what's referred to as "the fight or flight response" is regulated by the amygdala, a gland in the brain that's central to controlling emotions. In response to a threat, the amygdala triggers the release of steroids, including cortisol, known as the stress hormone. Also released are neurotransmitters like adrenaline, which may help shut down a part of our brain used for thinking clearly in addition to increasing our heart rate.

When we're doing serious exercises, the release of stress-related hormones can help us get the most out of our workout. And exercise is a stressful activity in that we're asking our muscles to respond to above-normal demands. The release of cortisol into our bloodstream can also be a warning, giving us notice we need to make a change. If you're in an argument, for example, and you feel your muscles tighten and you start sweating or your mouth gets dry, these are signs from your body that you need to resolve the issue quickly.

STRESS - WHAT IS IT?

Acute stress, or the body's reaction to an immediate threat, can have a negative impact. As long as the response is short and the body processes the cortisol, the long-term negative effects can be minimal. In the recovery state, our immune system, our hunger mechanism and our cardiovascular system — all of which respond to a threat — will return to normal.

If there are often-repeated incidents of acute stress, however, and if the body is constantly responding to a perceived threat, then stress can be very detrimental. It's for this reason some stress management techniques focus on helping individuals control the fight-or-flight response, and essentially try to eliminate the amygdala from the equation. Practitioners of these techniques believe that by approaching the stresses from an intellectual point of view, rather than an emotional one, we're better able to manage our body's reaction and thus avoid long-term damage.

Almost all of us have probably been told the best way to calm down in a stressful situation is to count to 10 and take deep breaths. The theory behind that advice is that by doing so we're sending more oxygen to the part of our brain that thinks logically and giving it time to respond so it can override the amygdala. But what happens when stress is chronic? How do our bodies react when we're always worried or always feeling overwhelmed?

If we go back to an analogy I used early on comparing the body to a car, then we can see living with chronic stress is like having your engine always revved up and ready to take off. Is it any wonder, then, that those suffering from chronic stress can't sleep?

If you're suffering from chronic stress, you're increasing your risk of getting sick. It's important you recognize the dangers of chronic stress and discuss the issue with your physician. While there are many techniques that can be used to help minimize stress, those who suffer from chronic stress might be encouraged by health-care professionals to make lifestyle changes.

Exercise and a healthy diet are as important to improving your response to stress as attitude and awareness. If you've taken steps to manage your chronic stress but still feel the effects — an inability to sleep well, clammy skin, sweating or constant edginess — see your doctor.

Remember, chronic stress and uncontrolled acute stress can cause long-term damage to your body.

CHAPTER 38

THE IMPORTANCE
OF MANAGING STRESS

For centuries people have recognized the connection between mental attitudes and health. Until fairly recently, those suffering from many illnesses would be sent to spas or vacation spots to relax and recover.

Today, as science and technology improve, researchers are discovering there's an even greater link between emotional attitude and illness. Thanks to modern science, stress – essentially a physiological or psychological response to anything perceived as a threat or as overwhelming – has now been identified as a contributing factor to many physical illnesses.

Recently, scientists have been able to draw a connection between stress and the effectiveness of the immune system, further strengthening the connection between chronic stress and increased susceptibility to everything from the common cold to serious diseases.

And there are strong indications stress is an important factor in aging, causing the release of free radicals that have been linked to cell damage.

There's also strong evidence to support the belief that reducing stress can help you eat better, sleep better and feel better both mentally and physically.

Doctors have been aware of the relationship between stress and heart disease for decades. A study in 2001 showed that reducing stress after a heart attack improved the prognosis for a successful long-term recovery.

Some researchers believe stress management programs might be as effective, if not more so, than exercise in preventing heart disease. Stress management programs might help reduce the risk of heart attacks by as much as 75 percent in people with heart disease.

As I've discovered, stress management techniques can also help you reduce your blood pressure and can be effective in preventing chronic headaches. According to the Centers for Disease Control in Atlanta, almost 85 percent of the deaths in people between 18 and 65 years of age are related to lifestyle. Stress is certainly a lifestyle factor.

THE IMPORTANCE
OF MANAGING STRESS

Stress and Related Illnesses

Among illnesses and medical problems that have been linked to stress are:

Heart Disease

Doctors say stress can be a major contributing factor in the creation of clogged arteries. The theory is that blood becomes stickier, perhaps in anticipation of injury, during the fight-or-flight response associated with stress. In addition, scientists believe cholesterol levels increase during stressful situations in response to body fat releases, and that stress can cause arteries to constrict. Stress is most certainly a factor in blood pressure increases in many people, and dozens of studies document the relationship between hypertension and heart disease.

Weight Gain and Diabetes

Obesity and diabetes have been linked to heart disease for decades, and the latest studies show the link is stronger than first believed. Now there's evidence both ailments are related to stress. So it makes sense that if you cut back the stress, you have a better chance of avoiding diabetes and obesity and thus a better chance of avoiding heart disease.

Cortisol has been linked to an increase in fat in the abdomen and may result in increased weight among healthy people during periods of high stress. In addition, stress-related hormones have been connected to increased cravings for sugar or salt, which could lead to overeating.

Researchers now say chronic stress can lead to the body's inability to effectively use insulin. When that happens, blood sugar regulation is impaired and that can lead to diabetes.

Strokes

Research, including a study detailed in the June 2003 issue of *Stroke* and supported by a Danish study, concluded that men with elevated blood pressure levels during stressful situations were at a higher risk for strokes than men not affected by stress. In addition, research on aging has shown stress can increase brain deterioration and the rate at which cells are destroyed.

THE IMPORTANCE
OF MANAGING STRESS

Memory Loss

A study conducted in December 2004 by researchers at Yale University confirmed there are brain chemicals linking stress to reduced reasoning functions in animals. That could mean chronic stress can impair new learning and contribute to short-term memory loss and the inability to concentrate or to verbalize thoughts. Research in which subjects were given cortisol showed those taking the steroid scored significantly worse on memory tests than those who were given a placebo.

Gastrointestinal Problems

Chronic stress has been linked to everything from a peptic ulcer to irritable bowel syndrome. Again, the culprit might be one of several hormones released during severely stressful situations that can lead to an increase in the digestive acids in the stomach. Many doctors believe flare-ups of illnesses such as ulcerative colitis and Crohn's disease can be triggered by stress.

Immune System Deficiencies

Research by the National Institute of Mental Health has suggested links between the immune system and the brain, further compounding the belief that chronic stress can lead to susceptibility to infections. The reason is that cortisol is used to suppress the immune system and thus reduces the number of white cells available to fight off infections.

Other Disorders

Over the years, there have been studies that clearly link chronic stress to pain and to everything from insomnia to irregularities in the reproductive system. There are also indications stress can trigger allergies and skin disorders and could even be related to loss of hair and teeth.

Knowing the severe impact stress has on your health, one has to wonder why anyone would continue to live with a chronic stressful condition. To maximize a healthy lifestyle, treating or managing stress is of critical importance.

CHAPTER 39

GOLF AND MANAGING STRESS

I love to golf. At least five days a week, weather permitting, I'm on the golf course playing with a group of buddies in friendly competition. On top of that, I'm usually at the driving range every day for half an hour or so, just hitting a bucket of balls.

Some might consider all of this part of their daily exercise routine, but I don't go along with that. To me, time on the course is a supplement to the exercise I need to be doing, not a replacement. My time on the course or at the range is mentally challenging and relatively stress free, and it keeps me out of the house.

Don't get me wrong. Golfing can be stressful, especially if I'm playing poorly. But the thing about golf or any competitive activity, whether it be cards or tennis, or bridge or bowling, is that it helps take your mind off situations that might be causing you stress.

Golfing is one way I manage stress, but I've found no matter who you are, there's probably an activity you enjoy enough so you focus your thoughts on what you're doing, not on your problems. This isn't rocket science and we're not breaking any new ground here. But sometimes we need to remind ourselves that playing, whether it's getting involved in a game or just doing crossword puzzles, can help us put the situations that stress us into their proper place.

Smart and innovative companies understand play is good for managing stress. It's not that unusual today to walk into a high-stress work environment and see a ping-pong table or pinball machine inside or a basketball net in the parking lot.

I read somewhere that Katie Couric, the host of NBC's *Today* show and a woman who appears to be constantly in motion, has a way of handling stress that could be a model for others. She has discovered that playing a game of Scrabble with friends, even when she's stuck in a hotel room, can help her find an oasis of relaxation in a hectic schedule and keep her mind off the pressing issues of the day. And that's good for her health, according to researchers who say Americans spend too much of their leisure time catching up on things they need to do and not enough time having fun.

Playing doesn't necessarily have to refer to a game. A friend of mine has a brother who begins playing a harmonica when he's stuck in traffic. By focusing on the music and not the traffic jam, he can take advantage of a found moment and use it to unwind.

For me, I've discovered that planning time to relax – making sure I have regularly scheduled golf games – helps keep the stress down. Of course, some stress comes from playing in competitive situations. But for me, no matter how poorly I'm playing, the stress that comes from golf is not even in the same league as the stress that comes from having to deal with difficult work or family decisions.

For one thing, I'm usually with friends on the golf course and there's always some friendly chatter. Golf is also relaxing because you're outdoors in the fresh air and generally in nice weather. It's a game I love because every day is different and challenging.

But the biggest benefit I've found from golf is I'm so focused on my next shot or the strategy I'm using in the game, it's impossible for me to think about anything else. When I'm playing golf, my mind is always on the game. Stress occurs when I miss a shot, but it's usually short-lived. And that's important.

Studies show most of the time when stress is involved in health-related problems, it's the kind of stress that occurs over long periods of time and just wears you down. Playing sports or participating in any competition offers you less stress for a shorter time, and a chance to focus so intently that things you worry about are eliminated from your head, at least temporarily.

One way to manage the stress on the golf course, and in any activity, is to set realistic expectations. I try not to set my expectations too high and that way it's easier for me to enjoy the game.

While getting involved in a competitive activity always helps me relieve stress, it might not be for everyone. Some folks may enjoy just going out and doing volunteer work or tinkering in their garage. Once again, that activity provides you with an opportunity to focus your energy and thoughts away from your problems, so it can help you better deal with stress. Leisure activity helps keep you active so your mind doesn't dwell on your problems.

GOLF AND MANAGING STRESS

Studies show that people who live longer always have a reason to get up in the morning. I honestly believe it's important to fill your days with interesting and challenging activities and do them in a way that causes as little stress as possible. So if you feel a little stressed, go out and play. Enjoy a game or read a book. Focus your energies away from what's driving you crazy and put your mind on activities that are meaningful and pleasurable. You'll find that a round of golf every now and then, a game of bridge or an engaging book can be good for your long-term health and enjoyable at the same time.

CHAPTER 40

LEARNING TO RELAX

It's a phrase we hear a lot, especially when we're in a stressful situation: "You just need to relax." The unsolicited advice often comes from a well-meaning friend. And that person is right. The problem is many of us don't know how to relax. While we think of things like watching a movie or television, spending time with friends or even spending the day on the golf course as relaxing, the truth is that relaxation comes from clearing your mind.

Real relaxation comes when we actually shut out information, in many ways closing our minds to outside stimuli, at least momentarily, and giving our minds a chance to take a break. When I play golf, I focus my attention and concentrate on all the factors that create a good golf shot and a satisfactory score. As a result, my thoughts are totally removed from my problems during that time.

And while many folks think they know how to relax, few really can shut off their minds even for a short while. Over the years, and with the help of techniques I learned at the Pritikin Longevity Center and from others in the field, I've learned how to really relax and close off my mind. I can actually lower my pulse rate and my metabolic rate by relaxing. There are others who have honed the ability to relax so fully that they can actually shut off their analytical thinking ability altogether. For me, by using imagery and breathing techniques, I can cut back on my thinking to a point where I'm unaware of what's going on around me.

I've already talked about imagery and deep breathing, but there are other techniques some people use very effectively. One of the most popular is meditation, a technique that's continuing to grow rapidly. We'll discuss that in this chapter, along with other techniques including yoga, tai chi and pet therapy.

Meditation

Once considered the relaxation technique of folks who were outside the mainstream, meditation has become more and more widely accepted as one of the best ways to relax. It's so popular, in fact, that physicians are recommending it as a way to reduce stress and help lessen the effects of stress-related medical problems, which by some estimates account for 60 percent of all doctor visits. Dr. Ornish is a big proponent of relaxation and years ago proved that diet, exercise and relaxation, including meditation and yoga, can reduce the buildup of plaque in the arteries.

In recent years, researchers have made great strides in understanding the connection between mind and body and now have a pretty good idea of how meditation affects the brain, as well as the rest of the body. According to a 2003 *Time* magazine article "The Science of Meditation," research shows regular meditation can help rewire the brain so the fight-or-flight response is much more subdued. Other research indicates activity in certain areas of the brain, responsible for receiving and processing information about outside stimuli, is greatly reduced, leaving the person who's meditating much better able to shut out the outside world. By rewiring the brain's reaction to certain stimuli and to the fight-or-flight response, meditation can have a positive impact on the actual health of an individual because the body will no longer release the stress-related hormones as quickly or as readily.

Recent studies have shown meditation can have a positive impact on everything from increasing the number of flu antibodies in the bloodstream to increasing the number of immune cells used to combat breast cancer. Millions of Americans are discovering that meditation is easy and doesn't have to be time-consuming. While the standard for the amount of time it takes for meditation to be effective is about 20 minutes, there are some who believe the same effect can be achieved in just eight minutes a day. Almost all who teach meditation agree the key is finding something on which to focus your mind.

To effectively meditate, you should start by finding a quiet place to sit, either on a cushion or on a chair, where you can essentially shut out the rest of the world. You can meditate with the lights on or off, although off is sometimes preferred, but you should close your eyes and make sure you're centered on the seat.

Once in position, you need to focus on a phrase or a word or even on your breathing and actually say the word or the phrase to yourself repeatedly. Although your attention will shift, you can easily bring it back by focusing on the word or phrase you selected.

LEARNING TO RELAX

Yoga

Like meditation, yoga is an effective way to help people relax. But unlike meditation, yoga adds the physical element, using body movement to help stretch muscles and enhance relaxation.

Along with meditation, Dr. Ornish linked yoga to better health through his study published in the *Journal of Cardiology* in 1998 that showed lower cholesterol levels among those who combined yoga with meditation, exercise and a healthy diet. He says the combination not only helps reduce the risk of heart attacks, it can also reduce the risk of prostate cancer and other illnesses.

The reason, many would argue, goes back to stress and to the fight-or-flight response. Yoga combines mental and physical techniques, along with deep breathing methods, to create the relaxation response. As a result, lower levels of stress hormones are injected into the bloodstream and many of the physical ailments associated with chronic stress either disappear or never show up in the first place.

Researchers believe yoga can have a positive impact on your immune system since it might help speed up the flow within the lymphatic system and help the body filter out impurities. Unlike meditation, yoga tends to be a more social activity and yoga classes and studios can be found just about everywhere. An estimated 15 million to 20 million people practice yoga in the United States. Because it involves varying degrees of stretching, yoga can be effective for seniors and many yoga classes are designed specifically for people over 55. You can find them by checking with your local community center.

Tai Chi

Tai chi is an ancient form of exercise that looks a lot like martial arts being performed in slow motion. Besides relaxing you, it can help you avoid falling because it improves balance. There's also some belief that tai chi can be useful in combating shingles. A study done by the Oregon Research Institute in July 2002 indicated those who benefited most from tai chi were older people who were in good health but inactive. By taking a regular tai chi class, those individuals had an opportunity to increase their movement and sharpen their mental focus as well.

Like yoga, tai chi continues to grow in popularity and classes are popping up just about everywhere. Although tai chi can be a group exercise, individuals are encouraged to proceed at their own pace. If you're a person who could benefit from easy movement and are looking for a way to relax, then perhaps tai chi is for you.

Pet Therapy

For many of us, the best way to really relax is to connect with a friend – one with four legs. One of the ways I relax is to spend some time with Houdini, my cat, who acquired his name by disappearing into the walls of my home three times in his first four days with me. I've come home after many a stressful day and sat down in my easy chair, and within a couple of minutes the cat has jumped up into my lap. Right away, I find myself stroking him or brushing him and the problems of the day just melt away.

Dog lovers will also tell you their pets help them relax by drawing the focus away from problems. A dog who wants to play with you and offers you unconditional love after you've been stuck in traffic for an hour can be just what you need to unwind.

The net effect, no matter whether you're dealing with a dog, cat or another pet, is that you get involved with the animal, and that involvement helps you keep your mind off your problems. In many ways, having the responsibility of taking care of another living creature that depends on you can prove to be very relaxing.

CHAPTER 41

STRESS AND SLEEP

Do you find yourself losing sleep over your problems?

Do you wake up in the middle of the night and find it hard to get back to sleep or have trouble falling asleep in the first place?

If so, you're not alone.

Millions of Americans have trouble sleeping at night. In fact, according to a January 2004 *Business Week* article titled "I Can't Sleep," 54 percent of people over age 55 report insomnia at least once a week. For me, getting a good night's sleep has always been difficult. It's often hard to turn off my thoughts and stop thinking about the things I need to do.

While there are a variety of reasons people can't sleep, there's now pretty strong evidence to link insomnia to stress. The bottom line is that stress could be at the root of your sleeplessness and you might never even suspect it. It's not just a matter of thoughts not letting you sleep. Research shows there's a physiological link between chronic and acute stress and a lack of sleep because of the way stress hormones can actually interfere with the body's ability to relax.

While stress can cause sleeplessness, a lack of sleep can also lead to more stress. The result is a vicious cycle that can lead to other physical ailments as well as accidents or other problems resulting from a lack of alertness. Studies have documented people who are overtired are also unable to think as clearly as those who get a good night's sleep.

There's a great toll on Americans as a result of sleep loss. Researchers have linked sleep loss in women to heart disease and have shown sleep loss can have a negative impact on the immune system. Sleep loss might also be connected to diabetes.

Studies have put a dollar amount on sleeplessness with some researchers estimating that sleep disorders cost Americans $45 billion annually in lost productivity, health-care costs and motor vehicle accidents. Researchers have proved sleep deprivation leads to mistakes. In a study at the University of Pennsylvania, researchers were able to determine people who got only six hours of sleep a day make 11 times as many mistakes as people who get eight hours of sleep.

As we make more mistakes, we're likely to be more stressed. Scientists have also been able to show that those who are stressed, or perceive themselves to be stressed, wake up more frequently than those who don't perceive themselves to be under stress.

Doctors have also determined those who are stressed may not get as deep a sleep as those who aren't feeling pressures. One reason might be the stress hormones found in high amounts in people suffering from chronic stress. Studies have shown many people suffering from chronic insomnia have high levels of cortisol and other stress-related hormones in their bodies, which means their bodies are always in the fight-or-flight mode. As a result, heart rate can be elevated and the nervous system might be affected, making it difficult to sleep.

The lack of sleep combined with the effects of chronic stress can negatively affect your physical well-being along with your mental health. But it's not just chronic stress that can create sleeplessness. Chances are if you've had a particularly rough day, you might have trouble taking your mind off your problems, and that can mean a sleepless night. Researchers believe acute stress, anxiety over too much to do or a specific problem can interfere with the activities of the involuntary nervous system and affect your sleep.

So what can you do if you can't sleep? For me, a series of relaxation techniques combined with deep breathing can be helpful. We've talked about my relaxation techniques in a previous chapter. In my case, the key is to take my mind off of problems or issues.

One way to do that is to focus on things that are mechanical. Counting sheep, for instance, might work for some people because it requires you to concentrate on the sheep, not your worries. For me, mechanical exercise is focused on relaxing my body, muscle by muscle.

The best thing to do, however, might be to address your problem right then and there. One friend of mine, for example, couldn't sleep because a work deadline was nearing and he was worried about meeting it. So instead of lying in bed and worrying, he got up and did some work on the project. He was so focused on the work that he was able to fall asleep while sitting at the computer. Of course, not everyone can so directly address the issues that are keeping them awake in the middle of the night. But you might find taking some sort of action beneficial.

Preparation is also important, and there are many basic steps you can take before you go to bed to help you sleep better. One of the best things you can do, according to some experts, is to get regular daily exercise. This will not only help you sleep, it will also help you relax. Exercise reduces stress hormones in your bloodstream. For many people, a good walk an hour or so after dinner can help.

Watching what you eat and drink before you go to bed can also have an impact on how well you sleep. Some sleep experts recommend you put at least two hours between the time you eat a meal and the time you go to bed. I try to put three or four hours in between. Obviously, you'll want to avoid coffee and other beverages or foods with caffeine and might also want to avoid large amounts of alcohol before you go to bed.

If work-related stress is at the core of your sleeplessness, you might want to try separating your bedroom from work. Sleep therapists often advise their clients not to take work with them to bed, and many suggest keeping the television and the computer out of the bedroom.

Another option, one that has worked for me but one I try to avoid, is taking medication that will help you doze off. If insomnia is an issue and if you have trouble beating it on your own, consult your physician.

Still, if stress or worries are keeping you awake, then you might want to get back to the basics of stress management. First, find a way to avoid the stressful situation. If that doesn't work, try refocusing your thoughts so you won't dwell on your worries.

CHAPTER 42

DOS AND DON'TS
FOR MANAGING STRESS

- Don't sweat the small stuff. One of the most basic theories of stress management is to know how to prioritize. Follow the Serenity Prayer, which says learn to accept things you cannot change, change those you can and recognize the difference.

- Don't underestimate stress. In my younger years, I was like most people and had very little understanding of how deadly stress can be. Some researchers estimate 60 percent of office visits to doctors are due to stress-related illnesses and believe stress can be a factor in just about every major ailment from heart disease to stomach problems.

- Do know when to walk away. Get out of stressful situations whenever possible. If the pressure gets to be too great, whether it's in dealing with a situation or a person, then find a way to leave.

- Don't be afraid to take time for yourself. Take a nap in the middle of the day if you're stressed. Or listen to music or read a book. Taking a step away from the stress will help you manage it better.

- Do make it a point to know your strengths and weaknesses. Be honest with yourself about what makes you stressed. If you know that getting stuck in traffic stresses you, take less-congested roads. If you know you don't handle deadlines well, start earlier.

DOS AND DON'TS
FOR MANAGING STRESS

- Do take a break from stress. The impact of the surge of hormones flooding your bloodstream during "fight or flight" reactions can have a devastating effect on your body if allowed to go on for long periods of time. Count to 10 and breathe deeply when things are getting rough. It will help you think better.

- Do learn some stress-reduction techniques. Breathing exercises, meditation, imagery and many other techniques can help you invoke the relaxation response, the perfect antidote to the fight-or-flight response.

- Don't be afraid to play. Go out on the golf course or tennis court. Play a round of canasta or bridge. Whatever it is you enjoy doing, do it and focus on it to the point where you take your mind off what's creating stress in your life.

- Don't forget to laugh. Humor can be valuable in helping you keep stress in check. Look for it and enjoy it. It's good for you.

- Do remember to exercise. Physical activity can be a positive kind of stress and can help your body prepare for stressful times.

PART V

TOBACCO, ALCOHOL AND DRUGS

CHAPTER 43

HARMFUL SUBSTANCES

Nowhere in this book is the importance of moderation and avoidance of harmful behavior more pronounced than in this section, which would be better titled: Don't Do It, Don't Overdo It and Do It Right.

The key messages in this section are that if you smoke, stop; if you consume alcoholic beverages, use moderation; and if you take prescription drugs, be sure you're taking them correctly. It goes without saying that taking illegal drugs or abusing prescription drugs is just bad behavior.

Smoking

Fortunately, smoking has never been a problem for me, since even during my years in the service I was able to avoid the lure of tobacco. But I know how enticing it was and I know, from my friends who smoke, how hard it is break the habit.

That's no excuse. Everyone knows how bad smoking is for you; it's well documented. Forget that you'll in all likelihood suffer harmful effects if you continue to use tobacco, and forget it might mean your later years will not be as enjoyable as they could be. Instead, think about what your smoking is doing to your loved ones. Second-hand smoke can create health problems in people who have never lit up a cigarette. And what sort of example are you setting for your children, siblings, parents and friends?

The impact of your smoking goes beyond physical damage. Chances are that because you smoke, you'll need some assistance from your family down the road. Do you really want to put your loved ones through the agony of seeing you suffer from the effects that come from a lifetime of smoking? There's also the financial impact of smoking. You're spending money that could be put to better use. According to the federal government, every pack of cigarettes sold costs the nation $7 in medical care and lost productivity. Each year, smoking costs the country an estimated $158 billion or about $3,400 per smoker.

Some of you out there who are still smoking might say, "It's too late now. I've been smoking for 20 years and the damage is already done." That's not necessarily so. At the Pritikin Longevity Center, I saw the dramatic scan images of the lungs of someone who had been smoking and then stopped. What I saw was a steady progression of the lungs getting clearer and clearer, turning from black to pink over a series of months. The truth is that quite a bit of the damage from smoking, especially the damage to the lungs, can be reversed within six months to a year.

Some smokers I know have said they'll quit when they're ready. Knowing what we know, realizing there are now many tools available to help you stop, why wouldn't you be ready now?

Alcohol

Unlike tobacco, there might be some health benefits to alcohol, especially wine. The key, obviously, is moderation. You probably know red wine, in moderation, is actually good for you because it contains lots of antioxidants. But you wouldn't want to start drinking red wine, or any wine for that matter, to improve your health. My advice is that if you're a regular wine drinker, then drinking a glass or two as often as daily should not be a problem. If you're not, I wouldn't start. Why take the chance of becoming an alcoholic or having a DUI incident?

Beer is also a favorite of many people and, again, in moderation it's not a problem. But one of the downsides to beer is that often people don't drink it in moderation. Another downside is that beer, even light beer, contains a lot of calories and can hinder weight-loss efforts.

Today beer and wine seem to be replacing mixed drinks as the alcoholic beverages of choice. The days of dad coming home and sipping a martini are dwindling. And that's a good thing. Obviously, hard liquor is hard on your system. Once again, one of the best reasons not to overindulge in alcohol is that it might stand in the way of your being healthy or even getting close to reaching your 100th birthday. Too much alcohol can impair your judgment, leading to accidents, and it can have a negative effect on your liver as well as on your circulatory system.

Drugs

When most of us think of drugs being dangerous, we tend to think of illegal substance abuse. But one of the biggest problems for seniors is that prescription drugs, those in your medicine cabinet, can be deadly if not taken properly. There are documented cases of people forgetting when they last took their medicine and ending up taking an extra dose, causing serious problems. There are also many cases of people forgetting to take their medication and not getting the benefit from it.

According to the AARP, a third of people taking prescription medications say they don't always tell their doctor about other medications they're already taking, and one in five people surveyed said they had a prescription from their doctor they never filled. The truth is that how we take our prescription drugs, and how serious we are about making sure we take our medications, can have as much of an impact on our health as how much we exercise and what we eat.

Taking medication properly is a must if you want to live to 100.

The wrong combination of drugs can be dangerous, even deadly, according to the book *Drug Interaction Facts*, edited by David S. Tatro, a drug information analyst. Some drugs and supplements can interact with other medications and nullify their effects. They can also reduce or increase the amount of other drugs in your system to dangerous levels. So it's a good idea to read the label warnings on all over-the-counter and prescription drugs, as well as on nutritional supplements. In addition, be sure to tell each of your doctors all of the medications you're taking, both prescription and over the counter, along with any supplements, including vitamins, minerals and herbs.

It's also important to make sure you take the medications as prescribed. A recent study by a team at the Health Institute at Tufts-New England Medical Center showed that two out of every five seniors don't follow their doctors' instructions. Some seniors said they didn't take their medicines because they didn't see benefits, they didn't like the side effects or the costs were prohibitive. If you're not taking your medicines as prescribed, consult your physician and see whether there are beneficial alternatives.

As far as other drugs, illegal drugs, avoidance is a must. Even if you believe marijuana should be legalized, you might want to look at the research that shows the long-term effects of marijuana on the lungs and the brain. Most illegal drugs, aside from hindering judgment, can play havoc with your body and cause you to land in jail. The best way to avoid complications is to avoid these drugs altogether, not only because they're illegal and unhealthy, but because many are also addictive.

CHAPTER 44

MY STORY CONCERNING ALCOHOL, TOBACCO AND MEDICATIONS

This is a chapter in which the contents will be more about what I don't do than what I do. I don't smoke and never have. I don't drink except for a glass of wine every so often. And I don't take illegal drugs or abuse legal drugs.

One of the things I do, however, is to make sure that when I take medications, I take them properly and in compliance with the instructions of my physician. Statistics show medication is often not taken properly by seniors who are either forgetful or trying to save money by cutting doses in half. And it's clear taking medications improperly can be dangerous and in some cases fatal.

As we get older, it's natural for us to forget things. Forgetting to take our medications or remembering whether we took them can be an important issue. I can tell you that even with the precautions I take, I have forgotten to take medications on a number of occasions. It's easy, especially if you're on vacation or you're distracted.

In my case, because my medications are generally in low doses and taken more as a preventive measure than anything else, missing a dose is not critical. For someone fighting a specific disease or chronic illness, though, missing a dose can be extremely dangerous.

How Do I Make Sure I Take My Medications?

I take my medications and vitamins with meals, except when other times are more appropriate. All of us remember to eat, so if we get into the habit of taking our medications with meals, we're less likely to forget. But to make sure I take the right pills at the right time, I package vitamins and prescriptions in small envelopes that are clearly marked for each meal.

Each month when I get my medications, I spend about an hour putting together 90 packets – three for each day. All of the packets marked a.m. are exactly the same and contain the medications and

221

vitamins I need to take in the morning. There are also packets marked for lunch and packets marked for the evening.

One of the best things about these packets is they're portable. If I'm going to a restaurant, I can take the packet with me and I don't have to worry about pulling a collection of pill bottles out of my pocket. The same thing goes for when I'm traveling. Instead of having to take lots of pill bottles, I take several days' worth of packets with me that are small and compact. If you decide to use this technique, you might even want to label them by the day of the week.

A Bit More About Smoking

During World War II, everyone around me was smoking. I was actually a little bit of an outcast because I didn't smoke. The truth is I had tried smoking, actually to appear older and better fit in with my friends. But when I tried to inhale I ended up choking and that was the end of my experience as a smoker. I never missed it and I've never, after that, had any desire to try smoking.

I believe my abstinence from tobacco might be one of the reasons I've made it this far. If you think about it, I was living a terribly unhealthy lifestyle with a lot of stress. Had I added smoking to the mix, who knows what might have happened?

Smoking is probably one of the worst things you can do to your body. Yes, it's linked to a variety of cancers. It's also a leading cause of death in this country – primarily due to heart disease – and of emphysema. Its impact on the cardiovascular system is debilitating because it constricts blood vessels and thickens the blood.

These days, I don't like to be around people who smoke – although if it weren't for my ex-wife's attempts to give up smoking, I wouldn't have gone to the Pritikin Longevity Center. Then I might not have made the changes that have dramatically improved my life.

Personally, I can't say enough about the negative impacts of smoking. I find it hard to understand why anyone would start smoking or continue smoking, knowing what we know today about its effects on the human body.

MY STORY CONCERNING ALCOHOL, TOBACCO AND MEDICATIONS

Alcohol

Alcohol is a different story. Frequently, I'm with people who enjoy a glass of wine with dinner and I occasionally share a glass with them. I rarely consume all of the wine in a glass. The few times I drank a full glass, it caused me to fall asleep – my tolerance for alcohol is that low.

The cost of wine is also something to consider when going out to dinner. Restaurants usually charge $5 to $15 for a glass of wine, and the price of a bottle at a restaurant is likely to be twice what I'd pay for it in the store. I've paid many a restaurant bill and noticed alcoholic drinks represented 40 percent of the total.

CHAPTER 45

DOS AND DON'TS OF TOBACCO, ALCOHOL AND DRUGS

- Don't smoke. If you do, now's the time to quit.

- Do use moderation if you drink.

- Do take your prescription medication as directed by your physician.

- Do develop a system for helping you remember to take your medications.

- Do be sure to tell all of your doctors what medications you're taking, both prescription drugs and over-the-counter medications.

- Don't use banned substances.

- Do avoid abusing legal medications.

PART VI

ACCIDENTS, INJURIES AND ILLNESSES

CHAPTER 46

AVOIDING HAZARDS

It is so easy to forget how many hazards we encounter in our daily activities – and how much we tend to overlook the consequences.

How many times have you walked into a dark room in your home without turning on the light? How often have you walked alone in an area where it would have been easy for you to lose your balance and fall? And when was the last time you visited a friend who had a head cold, knowing that catching it could create a problem for you but ignoring the risk?

The truth is that as we get older, we're more vulnerable to accidents, injuries and illnesses. Taking the right steps to prevent these can help us reach our goal of living to 100.

The first thing we need to do is to recognize hazards and make a commitment to avoid them. But we also need to understand our limitations. I certainly wouldn't want to discourage you from pursuing any potentially hazardous activity – skydiving or skiing, for example – if it's something you want to do and feel capable of doing. It's important to remember that as you age, though, your reactions are slower and your bones become more brittle and heal more slowly.

Chances are you won't recover as quickly from a fall on the slopes at 80 as you might from a skiing accident at age 50. And in some cases, there's a chance you might not recover from a fall at all. According to the National Safety Council, falls or complications resulting from falls are a leading cause of death among seniors – although, of course, most falls that claim the lives of seniors take place in the home rather than during sports activities.

In this section, I'll address falls and what you can do to prevent them. We'll also look at their financial impact. And I've already covered in great detail one of the best ways to prevent falls: through exercise.

But falls aren't the only hazards we face. Traffic accidents are also an issue, with drivers age 65 and older having higher crash-death rates per mile driven than all other age groups except teen drivers. Why is that?

AVOIDING HAZARDS

Although most drivers over 55 are probably skilled and competent behind the wheel, once our bodies age, our reflexes slow down and our vision and judgment become less sharp. Our bodies can't endure trauma as well as they could when we were younger.

What should you do? Should you stop driving? Not necessarily, but you might want to consider your limitations realistically and adjust accordingly. In this section, we'll look at driver-safety issues and discuss steps you can take to avoid accidents and make the roads safer for both yourself and other drivers.

Along with the slowing of our reflexes and the deterioration of our eyesight and hearing, those of us who are older may also experience a decline in the sharpness of our memory. For the most part, the natural loss of memory is not life-threatening, but there are situations where it's important to make sure you remember to take simple steps such as locking the front door, disconnecting appliances or turning off the stove before you go to bed. One simple step might be to put together a checklist you can use before you go to bed to help you remember daily routines.

Preventing injury might mean being cautious when we're out in public. As we get older, we're more vulnerable to predators who might be after a purse or a nice watch. What can you do to avoid becoming a victim of crime?

The best advice in this arena is usually available from your local police department, but common sense tells you to be aware of your surroundings and keep your car doors locked whenever possible. If you park far away from a building, make sure you're in an area that is well lighted. Some people park far away during the daytime to get exercise but come back to their car only to find it has gotten dark and their car is in an isolated area. Also, we recommend not leaving valuables on the front seat next to you, even when you're in the car, since criminals have figured out how to smash the passenger-side window and grab a purse before you even know what's happening.

One of the best ways to avoid accidents and injury or illness is to always be proactive. I can't say enough about the importance of having a complete physical examination at least once a year and taking your medications properly. I recommend flu and pneumonia shots at the appropriate times as well as any other preventive inoculations your doctor advises.

AVOIDING HAZARDS

It's also important to avoid catching a cold in the first place. Stay home if possible rather than visit a friend or loved one who's struggling with a head cold. In some cases a cold can lead to pneumonia. And if you do come in contact with someone who's sick, do your best to wash your hands frequently to keep germs from spreading. In fact, you should also do this when you're sick to help shorten the time you're exhibiting symptoms.

Injuries and illnesses can often be prevented with a minimal amount of sacrifice. What you need, more than anything, is an awareness of your surroundings and your limitations. And, of course, a little common sense.

CHAPTER 47

MY STORY OF PREVENTION

There's no doubt that eating right, exercising, keeping your weight down and avoiding all tobacco and excessive amounts of alcohol will help you live to 100.

Even people in perfect health, however, are not immune to injuries or to losing their lives in accidents. However, there are measures you can take to help ensure your safety. Many are just simple common-sense steps.

It's important to understand that we're aging, and as a result we need to be more careful and take fewer chances than we did before. In this section, we'll discuss simple actions you can take, such as wearing a seatbelt while in a car, that can help you avoid injury in an accident.

I want to take a minute to tell you about something interesting that happened to me while I was putting together this book. It will illustrate the importance of living healthy and the importance I place on being proactive with your health. It also highlights the need to have a checkup at least once a year.

In March 2004, just a few weeks short of my 80th birthday, one of the intense physicals I have twice a year led my doctor to ask for follow-up tests. In the course of listening to my heart, he heard a murmur he thought might have been attributed to mitral valve prolapse – a failure of the valve to close fully – that I knew I'd had all of my life. After doing the tests, the doctors discovered one of the struts that hold the valve in place was weakening and could create problems in the future. To repair the problem, doctors would have to perform open-heart surgery.

At this point I was feeling fine. Up until I visited the doctor, I was continuing my workout routine, including strength training. The concern, of course, was that the struts could give way and the valve would then fail.

After getting the diagnosis, I faced several options. The first was to do nothing other than keep an eye on the problem and check again in six months. I wasn't in any pain, my heart was in excellent condition and the weakened strut wasn't interfering with my lifestyle. I had two trips planned, which would have to be canceled if I chose to have surgery.

The second option was to go on the trips and then be tested again when I returned to see whether deterioration of the strut had progressed. If we then found a problem that interfered with my daily life, I'd need to take action.

Then there was a third option: undergo the highly invasive and somewhat risky surgery as soon as possible.

My choice – keep in mind I was nearly 80 years old at the time – was to go for the surgery. In making my decision, I took many factors into consideration. One was the recommendation of my physician. A key to his recommendation was that I was in very good physical condition.

One of the greatest benefits of living a healthy lifestyle is that, should you need medical care or surgery, your body will be better prepared to handle it. Because I've been doing most of the right things over the past 25 years, my risk was greatly reduced. My physicians told me that because I was in good health, it suggested only a 2 percent risk as opposed to a 15 percent to 20 percent risk other 80-year-olds might have faced. Had I been in poor health, the doctors might have suggested avoiding surgery altogether, not just putting it off temporarily, because of the danger involved.

The fact that I was in good shape also helped cut down on my recovery time. Although I was weak after the surgery, I was never in a great deal of pain, nor did I lose my appetite. I did, however, lose around 15 pounds and had to work hard to get the weight back, which I did. Within a few weeks of surgery, I was back walking at least two miles a day. Within a month, I was back on the exercise bike and lifting light weights.

Being in good health also helped reduce the emotional stress that can come with surgery. I was confident I could endure the surgery and as a result didn't worry as much as others my age might have. Had this happened back in the days when I was working long hours and not taking care of myself, this surgery might have been much more stressful and dangerous.

Another key factor in my decision to have the surgery was my desire to be proactive and to prevent major problems when at all possible. Had I waited, the struts might have collapsed and then I would have been in an emergency situation. By taking a proactive approach, I was able to avoid seeing the problem escalate into a more difficult situation. In essence, I minimized the risk.

Minimizing risk is something I try to do in my everyday life. Each of us faces risks on a daily basis, whether it's while we're driving or just walking down the street. By understanding our physical limitations, we might be better able to protect ourselves from the accidents that can get in the way of our living to 100. In the rest of this section, I'll talk about some of the steps I take, or in some cases don't take, to make sure I'm safe. And I'll share with you some ideas on how you can be proactive in avoiding accidents as well.

CHAPTER 48

AVOIDING FALLS

Think the ski slopes are more slippery than your stairs?

Think again.

According to national statistics, more people die each year from falls on stairs or steps than on ladders or through athletic activities such as tennis or skiing. In fact, according to research available from the National Safety Council, more than 50 percent of all falls occur in the home.

In 2001, according to one study, more than 1.6 million seniors were treated in emergency rooms for falls, with about a quarter of them requiring hospitalization.

While some of these falls might not be preventable, there are steps you can take to eliminate the vast majority of falls that could lead to your injury or death. At the same time, it's important that we not take the idea of fall prevention to extremes and forget to live our lives. Studies show about one in four seniors encounters a disabling fear of falling and restricts physical activity unnecessarily.

One of the goals of this chapter is to help you better understand the ramifications of falling when you're over age 55. At the same time, I hope to give you information that will help you avoid falls while continuing to maintain your confidence.

Because falls have such an impact on Americans, especially seniors, a vast amount of research has been conducted. Summaries of many of these studies can be found on the website of the National Center for Injury Prevention and Control, http://www.cdc.gov/ncipc.

Falls are the accidents that affect seniors the most, according to the center's Tool Kit to Prevent Senior Falls. Seniors are five times as likely to suffer an injury in a fall than from any other accident. Sadly, one in three people who fall will suffer severe or moderate injuries that can increase their chances of dying earlier.

Almost 90 percent of all broken bones in seniors, according to studies, are the result of falls. And the National Alliance to Prevent Falls as We Age reported that 50 percent of those who do fall do so repeatedly.

AVOIDING FALLS

What's the cost of all these falls? Well, according to studies outlined by the National Center for Injury Prevention and Control, the falls take their toll both physically and financially.

Those over 75 who suffer an injury in a fall are much more likely to be admitted to a long-term-care facility for a year or longer. Even those 20 years younger can be affected severely. The most-likely injuries sustained in a fall are fractures of the hip, back, pelvis and extremities such as the arm or the leg, as well as of the hand and the ankle.

Of those fractures, the one that has proved to be the most serious is a hip fracture, with studies showing this type of injury leads to more deaths and reduces the quality of life more than any other. In 1999 alone, hip fractures put 338,000 people in the hospital. Research shows hip fractures become more likely as we get older. People like me, in their 80s, are 10 percent to 15 percent more likely to suffer a broken hip than are people in their 60s.

The financial cost of all of this can be staggering. Researchers believe that by 2040, the cost of treating hip fractures and caring for those who suffer from them will reach $240 billion.

With the costs so high – and falls representing one more obstacle to our goal of living to 100 – it's important that we take steps, literally and figuratively, to avoid this type of injury. As I mentioned, one of the best things you can do to avoid a fall is to make sure you stay healthy. Regular exercise, especially improving lower body strength, can be a big plus and can help you maintain your balance. And when you're exercising, make sure you carry a cell phone or have someone with you, even if you're just taking a walk. It's also a good idea to walk on smooth surfaces.

Some researchers advocate tai chi, yoga and other forms of exercise that require balance. Consult your physician to make sure your medications don't create problems with balance or drowsiness that can lead to a fall. And while you're at it, why not get your hearing and your vision checked, since poor hearing and poor vision can certainly lead to accidents? Our ears, you may recall, play an important role in balance.

So what are some of the things you can do around your home to minimize your risk of falling? The first place to start is on the stairs and outdoor steps, if you have any. The National Safety Council recommends you have two handrails, if at all possible, and that you make sure the steps are high and wide enough. If there is carpeting on the steps, it

AVOIDING FALLS

shouldn't be torn or loose. And by all means, have a light switch at both the top and bottom of the stairs.

The bathroom is another important place to take precautions, and it's easy to do. Put no-slip mats on the shower floor. If you can, install grab bars next to the tub and the toilet.

Throughout the remainder of the house, you can improve safety by making sure there's proper lighting, that extension cords are not in your walking path, and that clutter is removed. Clean up spills right away. By removing obstacles inside, you can minimize the risk of a fall.

You need to be careful outside your home as well. Use common sense when you're outside and take precautions. If you're riding a bicycle, for instance, wear a helmet to protect yourself from head injuries.

CHAPTER 49

DRIVER SAFETY

Here's a fact: as we get older, most of us experience a reduction in our reflex response time and a loss of some portion of our senses. Our hearing might not be as good as it was when we were 20, and we might have trouble seeing at night. Obviously, those losses can have an impact on our driving ability, but that doesn't necessarily mean we should put away the car keys for good. Instead, we need to be aware of our limitations and not be afraid to face them realistically.

Seniors need to make their own decisions on what limits to put on their driving and when to stop getting behind the wheel. We all need to recognize the signs. The minute you sense you're not stopping quickly enough or that you're turning wider than you should, that's the time to consider putting limits on your driving. If you end up in a couple of minor traffic accidents within a short time, that could be a warning that a serious accident might occur in the future if you don't make some changes. Also, talk to your physician about your limitations and ask for advice on your driving abilities.

Remember, just because we're getting older doesn't mean we're not safe drivers. It just means we might be limited.

Although I'm 80, I continue to drive but I have restricted my time behind the wheel to short trips and daytime driving. Most of us, as a matter of fact, are driving smarter and safer as we get older. According to studies, seniors are more likely to wear seatbelts than any other age group except infants, we avoid driving in bad weather conditions, and we're less likely to drink and drive than other adults.

But we are also more likely to experience serious injury than younger drivers if we're involved in a crash. A 2004 study by the AAA Foundation for Traffic Safety shows drivers over age 65 are twice as likely to die in an accident than someone between 55 and 64. Drivers over 85 were nearly four times as likely to die in a crash.

That same study showed that lapses in perception – running a red light or not paying attention to a yield sign – were contributing factors in 60 percent of accidents involving drivers over 75. Impaired judgment, especially when making a left turn, also was cited by the study as an issue of concern for senior drivers. The chances of seniors over 65 getting into an accident when making a left turn were 25 percent greater than they were for most middle-age drivers, the study showed.

So what can we do to avoid becoming part of those grim statistics?

For me, the answer is to slow down a little, leave more space between my car and the vehicle in front of me, and always allow plenty of time to get where I'm going. When I'm taking a short trip on the highway, I always make it a point to stay to the right and to travel at about the speed limit. My goal is to drive at a pace where I have time to react to factors I can't control. Because not everyone realizes that driving fast will only save a few minutes on a trip while increasing risks, it's best to stay to the right.

When I'm driving, I always make it a point to leave early and drive at a reasonable speed so I don't have to hurry. By doing that, I can wait a few extra seconds when making that left turn and I can keep a steady pace.

Another positive step we can all take is to enroll in driver safety courses that are geared toward older adults. These courses, which are offered by safety organizations and police departments in many communities, help remind us we do have limitations and we can make adjustments that will decrease our chances of getting into an accident. Today, drivers who take these courses can get insurance discounts in more than 35 states.

We can help ensure our safety in the car by paying attention to maintenance. As we get older, the chances are reduced of our being able to fix a flat tire or push the car to the side of the road if we should stall. To avoid being in that position, we need to make sure we take care of our cars and, if you can afford it, buy a car that's known for reliability, dependability and safety.

All of us will experience a decline in our perception and motor skills as we age. By staying in good health, we can minimize the risk of being in an accident and suffering serious injury.

CHAPTER 50

DOS AND DON'TS FOR AVOIDING ACCIDENTS, INJURIES AND ILLNESSES

- Do recognize your limitations.

- Do install no-slip mats or surfaces in your bathtub and install grab bars near showers and toilets.

- Don't leave extension cords or clutter in places where they'll be in the way.

- Do fix loose steps.

- Do wear a helmet when bicycling.

- Do see your physician at least once a year.

- Don't knowingly put yourself in physical contact with people who have colds or other ailments that might be contagious.

- Do become aware of changes in your judgment, eyesight or hearing that could impair your ability to drive well.

- Don't follow the car in front of you too closely when driving.

- Do maintain an awareness of your surroundings in order to avoid becoming a crime victim.

PART VII
HEALTHY ATTITUDE

CHAPTER 51

STAYING POSITIVE

A healthy mind is just as important as a healthy body. Few of us would want to live to 100 if we were suffering from a disease such as Alzheimer's that robbed us of our cognitive functions. Over the years, considerable research has been done on the relationship between longevity and a healthy mindset. Most researchers will tell you the link is undeniable.

Studies have shown people who have a positive attitude about life, who stay busy and have something to look forward to, manage to live longer than those who don't. In her book *Too Busy To Count the Years*, author Suzanne Snyder Jacobson found that all of the people over age of 80 she wrote about had a routine and a reason to get up each morning. In fact, she found one woman who makes a cake every day and gives it away because that's her passion.

Magazine articles and several books written on longevity also attribute long life to an active mind combined with physical activity and a proper diet. I subscribe to that theory and believe it's important to keep your mind working all the time. A key aspect of having a healthy attitude is having a direction in your life.

All of us should set goals and we should have a passion about attaining them. What better time than now?

Over the course of our lives, most of us develop a list of things we'd love to do if we had the time and the money. In some cases, it's traveling and visiting places we always wanted to see. In other cases, it's going back to school and taking courses that can broaden our horizons. Now that most of us are retired, we have that time and we might also have the funds to pursue our dreams. Friends of mine keep their minds active through charity work and with visits to their grandchildren. For me, my involvement with numerous organizations, especially the Wellness Center at Oklahoma State University in Stillwater, is my passion and something I think about every day.

Generally, I'm thinking about what I can do to help improve the program at the Wellness Center so one day the school is recognized as having the healthiest student body in the country. While I'm involved in that project, I'd also like to see Stillwater recognized as the healthiest town in America.

The more we use the mind, the stronger it gets. In many cases, working on this book and sharing my successes regarding a healthy lifestyle have had a nourishing effect on my mind. Every day, I'm reading something in the paper about health and I'm cutting out articles.

Reading is critical to having a healthy mind. I read two newspapers each day: the local paper and *The Wall Street Journal*. On Sundays, I also read *The New York Times*. I stay informed, keep my intellect active and am able to contribute more to conversations about the events of the world. I also always have a book around to read.

Exercise is also important to having a healthy mind. A study conducted by the University of Illinois concluded exercise results in changes in the brain that improve our ability to make decisions and focus more clearly. Subjects in the study who walked briskly three times a week for six months did better than those who remained sedentary in tests that studied the ability to focus on specific tasks while disregarding irrelevant information. Researchers believe the changes in the brain that result from physical exercise will also lead to a decrease in cognitive decline that comes with the aging process.

One of the more fascinating parts of the study is that it supported two of the central theories in this book – that any effort toward a healthy lifestyle is better than none and that it's never too late to start.

In the study, researchers took 30 people with sedentary lifestyles between ages 60 and 79 and put half on a program involving a brisk walk for an hour three days a week. After six months, the people who took part in the walks had increased their cognitive skills by 11 percent, while those who didn't participate showed only a 2 percent increase in cognitive skills.

This study, and those that come in its wake, should eliminate any doubt about the benefits of exercise on the body and mind.

But there are other factors as well that can help us keep a healthy mind. One of those is maintaining our sense of perspective.

As we get older, we realize small things don't necessarily need to become bigger issues. By going with the flow more, by accepting what life throws at us, all of us can be happier. And I honestly believe the happier you are and the more goals you still have to achieve, the longer you'll live. Sure, all of us get down every now and then and we let things bother us for a lot longer than they should. But it's important to keep our troubles in perspective.

We can do that by becoming more accepting of what life deals us. Take positive steps toward resolving the issue, and reason through the problem.

If you keep your brain active and your body healthy, who knows what brilliance you might project at age 100?

CHAPTER 52

DOS AND DON'TS OF A HEALTHY ATTITUDE

- Do set goals and be passionate about achieving them.

- Do keep your mind active by reading, playing cards, playing golf or through any other game or activity that requires thought.

- Don't dwell on the negative but instead try to look at the positive side of things.

- Do remember exercise is good for your mind as well as your body.

- Don't lose your sense of perspective and allow small problems to become big ones.

- Do take positive steps toward resolving problems and reasoning through issues.

PART VIII

THE SERETEAN MEAL PLAN
AND RECIPES

BUD'S 7-DAY MEAL PLAN

I have a meal plan that is similar in some respects every day but also offers me a wide variety of healthy and delicious foods. Here's an example of one of my weekly menus. All of the recipes listed here are included later in this section.

Day 1

Breakfast: 4 ounces orange juice
1/2 cup Irish oatmeal with raisins and skim milk
1 slice whole grain toast
1 tablespoon non-fat yogurt cheese

Snack: 1 cup watermelon

Lunch: 1 cup lentil soup
4 ounces turkey burger with sautéed onions
1/2 cup Southern Salad
Roasted potato skin wedges
6 ounces grape juice

Snack: 1 cup non-fat cottage cheese, with
1/4 cup non-fat sour cream and 1/4 cup blueberries

Dinner: 2 cups fat-free Caesar salad
6 ounces grilled salmon with
2 tablespoons cucumber dill sauce
Baked sweet potato
1/2 cup spinach with garlic
6 ounces apple cranberry crumble
1 cup green tea

Snack: 3 ounces trail mix and 1 fat-free, sugar-free frozen fudge bar

244

BUD'S 7-DAY MEAL PLAN

Day 2

Breakfast: 4 ounces orange juice
1/2 cup Irish oatmeal with raisins and skim milk

Snack: 2 slices whole-grain raisin-walnut toast
1 ounce non-fat yogurt cheese
6 ounces hot skim milk

Lunch: 1 cup green split-pea soup
3 slices gourmet vegetable pizza
1 cup cantaloupe
6 ounces apple juice

Snack: 1 cup honeydew melon, 3 fat-free Fig Newtons

Dinner: 2 cups mixed salad with ginger dressing
6 ounces steamed sea bass with Asian sauce
1 cup spinach
1/2 cup carrots
1/2 cup basmati rice
1 cup fat-free, sugar-free blueberry frozen yogurt
1 cup green tea

Snack: Romanian polenta with non-fat sour cream

Day 3

Breakfast: 4 ounces orange juice
1/2 cup Irish oatmeal with raisins and skim milk

Snack: 1/2 cup stewed prunes

Lunch: 1 cup vegetable soup
Romanian eggs with tomatoes and onions
1 slice whole-grain toast
3 ounces Southern Salad
1 cup mixed berries

BUD'S 7-DAY MEAL PLAN

Snack: 1 baked apple, 4 graham crackers

Dinner: 2 cups fat-free Caesar salad
            1 cup whole-wheat pasta
            2 turkey meatballs with marinara sauce
            1/2 cup spinach with garlic
            1/2 cup sautéed red, green and yellow peppers
            6 ounces low-fat, sugar-free cheesecake with raspberry coulis
            1 cup green tea

Snack: 3 ounces trail mix, 3 fat-free Fig Newtons

Day 4

Breakfast: 4 ounces orange juice
            1/2 cup Irish oatmeal with raisins and skim milk

Snack: 2 slices whole-grain raisin-walnut toast
            1 ounce yogurt cheese
            6 ounces hot skim milk

Lunch: 1 cup onion soup
            1 cup Cowboy Chili
            1 cup wild and brown rice pilaf
            1 cup golden pineapple

Snack: 1 cup non-fat cottage cheese
            1/4 cup non-fat sour cream
            1/2 sliced banana

Dinner: 1 cup Southern Salad
            6 ounces balsamic chicken
            1 cup vegetable couscous
            1 cup roasted vegetable medley
            6 ounces peach crumble
            1 cup green tea

Snack: 1 cup fat-free, sugar-free frozen yogurt

BUD'S 7-DAY MEAL PLAN

Day 5

Breakfast: 4 ounces orange juice
1/2 cup Irish oatmeal with raisins and skim milk

Snack: 4 ounces applesauce with stewed berries

Lunch: 1 cup golden pea soup
2 salmon fritters (6 ounces)
1 cup Southern Salad
1 cup cantaloupe

Snack: 5 ounces Romanian polenta with non-fat sour cream

Dinner: 2 cups field greens salad with raspberry vinaigrette
6 ounces meatloaf with 2 ounces mushroom gravy
1/2 cup whipped sweet potato
1 cup herb-crusted broccoli and cauliflower
6 ounces apple-cranberry crumble
1 cup green tea

Snack: 3 ounces trail mix, 1 fat-free, sugar-free fudge ice cream bar

Day 6

Breakfast: 4 ounces orange juice
1/2 cup Irish oatmeal with raisins and skim milk

Snack: 2 slices whole-grain toast
1 ounce yogurt cheese
6 ounces hot skim milk

Lunch: 1 cup garbanzo bean soup
1 cup saffron pasta with veggies
1 cup mixed fruit

Snack: 1 apple and 3 ounces salt-free nuts

Dinner:	2 cups spring mix salad with balsamic Italian dressing
	6 ounces roasted chicken
	1/2 cup bread stuffing
	1/4 cup cranberry sauce
	1/2 cup French green beans almondine
	1/2 cup carrots
	1/2 cup light custard with 1/2 cup mixed berries
	1 cup green tea
Snack:	3 ounces trail mix, 3 fat-free Fig Newtons

Day 7

Breakfast:	4 ounces orange juice
	1/2 cup Irish oatmeal with raisins and skim milk
Snack:	1 cup Total cereal with 1/4 cup skim milk
	and 1/4 cup blueberries
Lunch:	1 cup white bean and spinach soup
	6 ounces chicken or salmon salad
	1/2 cup of fat-free coleslaw
	1 cup watermelon
Snack:	1 cup stewed fruit
Dinner:	2 cups fat-free Caesar salad
	6 ounces vegetable lasagna
	1 baked tomato
	1 cup broccoli and carrots
	6-ounce slice double-layer raspberry chocolate cake
	1 cup green tea
Snack:	1 cup mixed berries

HEALTHY RECIPES

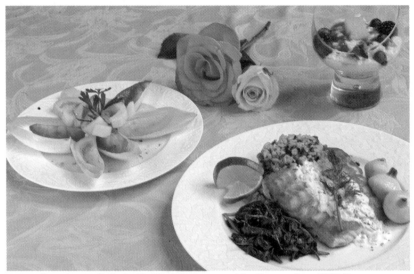

Southern Salad, Grilled Salmon with Cucumber Dill Sauce,
Wild and Brown Rice Pilaf, Spinach with Garlic,
and Light Custard with Berries

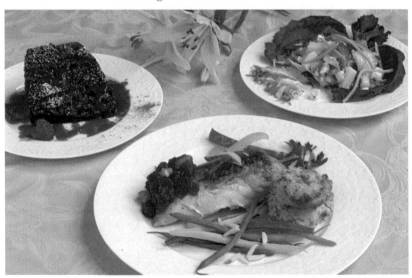

Chicken Salad, Roast Chicken with Cranberry Sauce,
Bread Stuffing, French Green Beans Almondine, and
Double-layer Raspberry Chocolate Cake

TABLE OF CONTENTS

SALADS AND SALAD DRESSINGS

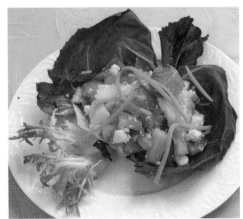

Chicken Salad

Southern Salad

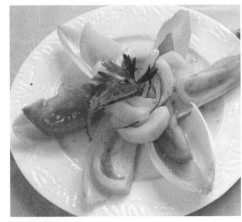

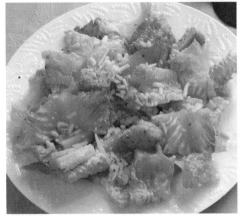

Caesar Salad

SALADS

Chicken Salad
Serves 4

2 six-ounce grilled chicken breasts (small-diced)
1/4 cup minced red onion (optional)
1/4 cup minced celery
2 tablespoons chopped walnuts
1 tablespoon dried cranberries
2 tablespoons Miracle Whip (fat-free)
1 teaspoon Dijon mustard
1 teaspoon chopped rosemary
Pinch of salt and pepper

Method:
Mix together all ingredients and chill for 1 hour.

Suggestion: serve in halved whole-wheat pita bread, or scoop on top of a mixed salad with fat-free Italian dressing.

Coleslaw
Serves 4

2 cups shredded green cabbage
1 cup shredded red cabbage
1 cup shredded carrots
1 teaspoon celery seed
1 tablespoon Splenda sweetener
2 tablespoons Miracle Whip (fat-free)
1 tablespoon rice vinegar

Method:
1. In a medium bowl, toss together all of the ingredients.
2. Refrigerate for 1 hour.

SALADS

Greek Salad
Serves 4

1 cup shredded carrots
2 cups spring salad mix lettuce, chopped
1 cup romaine lettuce, chopped
1 tomato, chopped
1 cucumber, seeded and chopped
1 ounce Greek black olives, pitted and halved
1 ounce green olives, pitted and halved
2 ounces reduced-fat feta cheese, crumbled
1 tablespoon reduced-fat Parmesan cheese

Dressing:
1 tablespoon balsamic vinegar
1 tablespoon Dijon mustard
1 tablespoon virgin olive oil
1 tablespoon fresh chopped basil
1/2 teaspoon black pepper
Pinch of salt

Method:
1. Chop all ingredients and place in large salad bowl.
2. Mix dressing separately.
3. Drizzle dressing on top.
4. Toss.
5. Refrigerate for one hour and serve.

Salmon Salad
Serves 6

1 can (16-oz.) red salmon (drained and center bone removed)
1/4 cup chopped scallions
1 tablespoon chopped fresh dill
1 tablespoon chopped celery
2 tablespoons Miracle Whip (fat-free)
Pinch of salt and pepper

Method:
1. Flake salmon.
2. Mix with remaining ingredients into a bowl.

Southern Salad
Serves 4

1 cup diced tomato
1 cup diced cucumber
1/2 cup sliced red onion

Marinade:
1/4 cup red wine vinegar
2 tablespoons Splenda sweetener
1 ounce water
Pinch of salt and pepper
1 tablespoon olive oil

Method:
1. Place tomato, cucumber and onion into a medium bowl with the marinade.
2. Cover the bowl and let stand in the refrigerator for 1 hour.

SALAD DRESSINGS

Balsamic Italian Dressing
Serves 4

1/2 cup balsamic vinegar
1 tablespoon Dijon mustard
1 teaspoon roasted garlic, minced
2 teaspoons Splenda sweetener
1 tablespoon chopped basil
1 tablespoon chopped Italian parsley
1/4 cup olive oil

Method:
1. In medium aluminum bowl, whisk together vinegar, mustard, garlic, Splenda and herbs.
2. Slowly whisk in olive oil to prevent separation.

Caesar Dressing
Serves 4

2 tablespoons Dijon mustard
2 tablespoons white balsamic vinegar
2 tablespoons reduced-fat Parmesan cheese
1 teaspoon white wine Worcestershire sauce
1 egg white
Pinch of salt and pepper

Method:
1. In a medium bowl, whisk together all ingredients except the egg whites.
2. Slowly fold in the egg white.

Ginger Dressing
Serves 4

1/2 cup grated carrot
1 tablespoon finely chopped ginger
1/2 cup rice vinegar
1 tablespoon low-sodium soy sauce
2 tablespoons Splenda sweetener
1/4 cup toasted-sesame oil

Method:
1. Place all ingredients except the sesame oil into a blender and mix.
2. Slowly add the sesame oil into the blender on low speed for 1 minute to prevent separation.

Honey Mustard Dressing
Serves 4

2 tablespoons Dijon mustard
1 tablespoon honey
1 tablespoon white balsamic vinegar
1 tablespoon chopped basil
1 tablespoon chopped dill
1 tablespoon chopped parsley
1 tablespoon olive oil

Method:
1. In a medium aluminum bowl, whisk together all ingredients except the olive oil.
2. Slowly whisk in the olive oil to avoid separation.

Raspberry Vinaigrette
Serves 4

1/2 cup raspberry vinegar
1/2 cup fresh raspberries
1 tablespoon Splenda sweetener
Pinch of salt and pepper
1/4 cup olive oil

Method:
1. Place all ingredients except the olive oil into a blender and mix.
2. Slowly add olive oil into the blender on low speed for 1 minute to prevent separation.

SOUPS

Garbanzo Bean Soup
Serves 4

4 cups water
1 can (16 ounces) garbanzo beans (rinsed)
1/2 cup diced celery
1/2 cup peeled and diced potato
1/4 cup diced carrot
1 peeled and minced shallot
1/2 cup chopped tomato
1 teaspoon minced garlic
1/2 cup corn kernels
1/2 teaspoon cayenne pepper
2 teaspoons low-sodium soy sauce
1 tablespoon crumbled fresh parsley
2 tablespoons chopped scallion

Method:
1. In a medium pot, bring water to a boil. Add all ingredients except parsley and scallion.
2. Lower temperature to medium and cook for 20 minutes, stirring occasionally.
3. Add parsley and scallion.

Golden Pea Soup
Serves 4

6 cups water
1 cup golden split peas
1/2 cup diced carrot
1/2 cup diced celery
1/2 cup diced sweet potato
1 teaspoon olive oil
1 shallot, minced
1 teaspoon minced garlic
1 teaspoon minced ginger
Pinch of salt and pepper
1 teaspoon fresh thyme

Method:
1. In a medium pot, bring water to a boil.
2. Add all ingredients except the thyme.
3. Lower temperature to medium, stirring the mixture occasionally. Cook for 30 minutes.
4. When the pea soup starts to form a fairly thick consistency, add the thyme and serve.

Green Split-pea Soup
Serves 4

1 teaspoon olive oil
1/2 cup chopped onion
1/2 cup diced carrot
1/4 cup diced celery
1 cup dried green split peas (rinsed)
6 cups water
1 clove garlic, minced
1 teaspoon cumin
1/2 teaspoon cayenne pepper
2 teaspoons low-sodium soy sauce

Method:
1. Heat pot to medium temperature.
2. Add oil. Cook onion, carrot and celery until translucent. Stir frequently.
3. Add remaining ingredients. Cook uncovered for 30 minutes, stirring occasionally.

Note: If soup gets too thick, add 1 cup dry sherry or water and stir.

Lentil Soup
Serves 4

6 cups water
1 teaspoon minced ginger
1 cup lentils
1/2 cup diced potato
1/4 cup chopped onion
1/4 cup chopped tomato
1/4 cup diced carrot
1 teaspoon cumin
1 teaspoon curry
Pinch of salt and pepper
1 teaspoon Dijon mustard
1 teaspoon olive oil
2 tablespoons fresh parsley, chopped
1 tablespoon balsamic vinegar

Method:
1. In a medium pot, bring water to a boil. Add all ingredients except parsley and vinegar.
2. Lower temperature and cook uncovered, stirring occasionally.
3. When soup starts to thicken, add parsley and vinegar. Stir.
4. Cook until slightly thick, approximately 30 minutes.

Onion Soup
Serves 4

4 cups water
1 Vidalia onion, sliced
1 red potato, cut up
1/2 teaspoon roasted garlic
2 teaspoons olive oil
1 red onion, sliced
1 teaspoon Dijon mustard
Pinch of salt and pepper
1 teaspoon reduced-fat Parmesan cheese

Method:
1. In medium-sized pot, bring water to a boil. Add Vidalia onion, potato and garlic to the water.
2. Reduce temperature to medium. Cook for 20 minutes, stirring occasionally.
3. Meanwhile, heat oil in medium skillet. Add red onion and sauté until translucent. Lower temperature and continuing cooking until caramelized. Set aside.
4. When potato pieces are tender, blend the cooked mixture until smooth.
5. Add the caramelized onion, mustard, salt and pepper. Stir.
6. Sprinkle with Parmesan cheese and serve.

Vegetable Soup
Serves 4

6 cups water
1/4 cup broccoli florets
1/4 cup diced carrot
1/4 cup diced celery
1/4 cup diced onion
1/4 cup cauliflower florets
1/4 cup shredded cabbage
1/4 cup diced tomato
1/4 cup chopped asparagus
1/2 cup red potato, peeled and diced
1 teaspoon Dijon mustard
1/2 teaspoon saffron
Pinch of salt and pepper

Method:
1. In a medium pot, heat water until boiling. Lower temperature to medium and add all ingredients.
2. Cook for 20 minutes, stirring occasionally.

White Beans and Spinach Soup
Serves 4

4 cups water
1 can cannelloni beans
1/2 cup peeled and diced red potato
1/4 cup chopped onion
1/4 cup diced red pepper
1/2 cup chopped tomato
1/4 cup diced carrot
Pinch of salt and pepper
3 cups fresh, cleaned spinach

Method:
1. In a medium pot, bring water to a boil. Add all ingredients except the spinach.
2. Lower temperature. Cook for 20 minutes, stirring occasionally.
3. Add spinach, stir and cook for an additional 5 minutes.

Note: Spinach should be bright green when done.

SAUCES AND GRAVIES

Asian Sauce
Serves 4

2 tablespoons low-sodium soy sauce
1/4 cup rice vinegar
1/4 cup dry sherry
2 tablespoons toasted-sesame oil
1 tablespoon fresh grated ginger
1 tablespoon chopped scallion

Method:
Mix together all ingredients and place in refrigerator for 1 hour.

Note: Use with Steamed Sea Bass and Spinach (see recipe).

Cranberry Sauce
Serves 4

1/2 can whole-fruit cranberry sauce
1 navel orange, diced
1/4 cup chopped walnuts
1 tablespoon freshly squeezed orange juice
1/2 teaspoon zest of lemon

Method:
In a medium bowl, mix all ingredients together.

Note: Serve with roast chicken or turkey.

Marinara Sauce
Serves 6

5 vine-ripened tomatoes, diced
1/2 cup coarsely chopped onion
2 teaspoons minced garlic
1 tablespoon tomato paste
1 teaspoon Splenda sweetener
1/2 cup red wine
1 teaspoon crushed red pepper
2 tablespoons fresh chopped basil

Method:
1. Heat a medium pot; add all ingredients except the basil. Cook covered at medium heat for 20 minutes.
2. Lower temperature to simmer, remove cover and add basil, stir.
3. Remove from heat, serve with pasta.

Mushroom Gravy
Serves 8

1 cup chicken broth, non-fat, low-sodium
1 cup dry sherry
2 cups sliced shitake mushrooms
1 cup chopped oyster mushrooms
1/4 cup minced red pepper
1/4 cup minced onion
1/4 cup chopped scallion
2 teaspoons low-sodium soy sauce
1 teaspoon Dijon mustard
1 teaspoon crushed roasted garlic
2 tablespoons crumbled fresh Italian parsley

Method:
1. In a medium saucepan, heat chicken broth and sherry until mixture boils, then lower heat to simmer.
2. Add remaining ingredients. Cook for 15 minutes or until desired thickness is reached.

Note: Serve with Turkey Meatballs (see recipe).

ENTREES

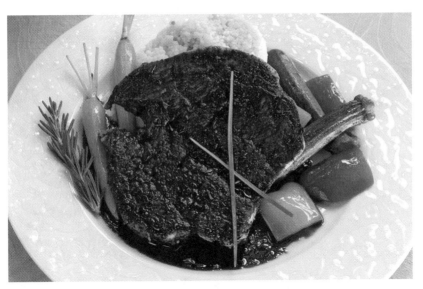

Balsamic Chicken, Romanian Polenta and Roasted Vegetable Medley

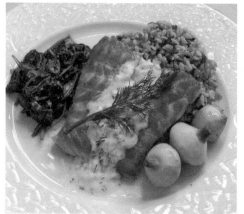

Grilled Salmon with
Cucumber Dill Sauce,
Wild and Brown Rice Pilaf,
and Spinach with Garlic

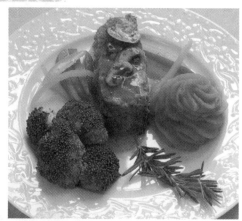

Meat Loaf with
Mushroom Gravy,
Whipped Sweet Potatoes,
and Herb-crusted Broccoli

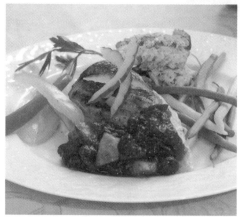

Roast Chicken with
Cranberry Sauce,
Bread Stuffing, and
French Green Beans
Almondine

Balsamic Chicken
Serves 4

4 six-ounce skinless boneless chicken breasts (pounded)
2 tablespoons olive oil
2 tablespoons chopped thyme
2 tablespoons chopped rosemary
1 tablespoon chopped basil
1 tablespoon chopped Italian parsley
Pinch of salt and pepper
8 ounces balsamic vinegar

Method:
1. In a large aluminum bowl, mix all ingredients except vinegar. Evenly coat each chicken breast with the sauce mixture.
2. Marinate chicken in refrigerator for 1 hour. Turn frequently.
3. Preheat oven to 400° F.
4. Place chicken in cast-iron skillet and cook at 400° Fahrenheit for 16 minutes. Turn once.
5. Heat a medium saucepan. Add vinegar and cook at medium temperature until vinegar thickens.
6. Drizzle vinegar reduction over the chicken.

Suggestion: chicken breasts can be dipped into the sauce to coat completely.

Cowboy Chili
Serves 2

8 ounces extra-lean (3% fat) ground round
1 teaspoon roasted garlic
4 ounces canned chili beans (rinsed)
2 tablespoons diced carrot
2 tablespoons diced celery
2 tablespoons chopped red onion
1/4 cup diced red pepper
1/4 cup diced green pepper
1 cup Enrico's low-sodium salsa
1 teaspoon low-sodium soy sauce
1 teaspoon chili powder
1 teaspoon cumin
1/2 teaspoon cayenne pepper
1 cup white wine

Method:
1. In a medium nonstick heated skillet, add ground round and stir until browned.
2. Add remaining ingredients. Stir occasionally and cook for 20 minutes.
3. When chili is thick, serve.

Gourmet Vegetable Pizza
Serves 2

1 French Meadow sourdough pizza crust
2 tablespoons Contadina tomato paste
1/4 cup red pepper
1/4 cup green pepper
1/4 cup yellow pepper
1/4 cup onion, chopped
1/4 cup carrot, chopped
1/4 cup broccoli florets
1/4 cup sliced mushrooms
1/4 cup tomato, chopped
1 teaspoon roasted garlic
1 tablespoon olive oil
1 teaspoon oregano
1/2 teaspoon crushed red pepper
1 teaspoon Italian seasoning
1/2 cup part-skim milk mozzarella cheese

Method:
1. Preheat oven to 375° Fahrenheit.
2. Spread tomato paste evenly on pizza crust.
3. Sauté the vegetables, tomato and garlic with the olive oil in a medium, heated skillet.
4. Place the sautéed ingredients on the pizza crust, over the tomato paste.
5. Top with spices and cheese.
6. Bake at 375° for 15 minutes.

ENTREES

Grilled Salmon with Cucumber Dill Sauce
Serves 6

24 ounces salmon fillets (Remove skin and cut into 6 portions)

Sauce:
In a medium bowl, mix:
6 ounces non-fat sour cream
1/2 cup seeded, chopped cucumber
1 tablespoon Dijon mustard
1 teaspoon fresh lemon juice
2 tablespoons fresh, chopped dill
Pinch of salt and pepper
Cover and refrigerate for 1 hour.

Method:
1. Heat a nonstick grill pan, to medium temperature and coat with cooking spray.
2. Cook fish for 3 minutes on each side or until grill marks form.
3. Top with cucumber dill sauce and serve.

Healthy Franks and Beans
Serves 2

2 fat-free turkey dogs
4 ounces vegetarian baked beans (canned)
1 teaspoon roasted garlic
1 tablespoon finely chopped onion

Method:
1. Heat a nonstick grill pan to medium temperature. Coat pan with cooking spray.
2. Cook turkey dogs on grill pan for 5 minutes (until grill marks show). Set aside.
3. Heat a small pot. Add beans, onion and garlic. Cook at medium temperature for 7 minutes. Transfer to serving bowls and top with turkey dogs.
4. Serve with sauerkraut.

Meat Loaf
Serves 6

1 pound extra-lean (3% fat) ground round
2 egg whites
1/4 cup oats
1/4 cup whole-wheat pita crumbs
1 teaspoon Italian seasoning
1 tablespoon reduced-fat Parmesan cheese
1 tablespoon Dijon mustard
1/2 cup minced celery
1/2 cup minced carrot
1 minced shallot
2 tablespoons chopped Italian parsley
Pinch of celery seed, salt and pepper
1 cup Marinara Sauce (See Marinara Sauce recipe.)

Method:
1. Preheat oven to 350° Fahrenheit.
2. In a large bowl, mix together all ingredients except the marinara sauce.
3. Place the mixture into a coated Pyrex loaf pan, smoothing even with a fork.
4. Pour the marinara sauce over the top of the meat loaf. Cover loaf with aluminum foil formed into a tent shape.
5. Bake at 350° for 40 minutes.

Note: serve with Mushroom Gravy (see recipe).

ENTREES

Roast Chicken
Serves 4

1 five-pound roasting chicken, cleaned, wing tips cut off, and pierced all
   over with fork
1 tablespoon I Can't Believe It's Not Butter
1 teaspoon Italian seasoning
1 teaspoon paprika
Pinch of salt and pepper

Method:
1. Preheat oven to 350° Fahrenheit.
2. Melt butter in small saucepan, adding the seasonings as you stir.
3. Coat chicken with seasonings (under the skin and inside the cavity).
4. Place seasoned chicken in roasting pan. Cover with foil and bake at
    350° for 1 hour. Baste chicken frequently.
5. Remove foil the last 20 minutes of cooking.
6. Remove skin and serve.

ENTREES

Romanian Eggs
Serves 2

1 whole egg
5 ounces Egg Beaters
1 tablespoon fat-free sour cream
1/4 cup finely chopped tomato
1/4 teaspoon cayenne pepper
Pinch of salt
1 teaspoon olive oil
1/4 cup finely chopped onion

Method:
1. In a medium aluminum bowl, gently whip all ingredients together except the onion. Set egg mixture aside.
2. In a medium skillet, heat oil.
3. Add onion to skillet and stir. Cook until onion is translucent.
4. Add onion to egg mixture in bowl.
5. Heat a medium skillet. Coat with cooking spray, add egg mixture and gently stir until scrambled.
6. Serve with whole-grain toast and yogurt cheese.

Salmon Fritters
Serves 2

1 can (6 ounces) red salmon (discard bones)
2 tablespoons minced onion
4 tablespoons minced celery
1 teaspoon chopped fresh dill
1 teaspoon salt-free ketchup
Pinch of salt and pepper
2 egg whites
1/2 cup whole-wheat pita bread crumbs

Method:
1. Mix all ingredients together and form fritters.
2. Heat a medium nonstick skillet. Coat with cooking spray.
3. Cook fritters in skillet at medium heat for 8 minutes, turning once.

Steamed Sea Bass and Spinach
Serves 4

4 six-ounce sea bass fillets
1/2 cup Asian Sauce (See Asian Sauce recipe.)
1 pound cleaned spinach
1 cup water
1 teaspoon lime juice

Method:
1. Marinate fish in Asian Sauce for 1 hour in refrigerator.
2. Remove fish from marinade and place in a large steamer basket. Set aside the remaining marinade.
3. Top fish with spinach.
4. Mix the water with the remaining marinade and lime juice. Pour into a large pot.
5. Place steamer basket with fish and spinach into the pot. Cover.
6. Cook over medium heat until steaming, about 5 minutes.

Turkey Burgers
Serves 2

6 ounces ground turkey breast
2 tablespoons minced celery
2 tablespoons minced carrot
1 tablespoon minced onion
1 teaspoon reduced-fat Parmesan cheese
1 teaspoon Dijon mustard
1 teaspoon no-salt ketchup
1 teaspoon low-sodium soy sauce
1/2 cup ground whole-wheat pita bread
2 egg whites

Method:
1. Mix together all ingredients, folding in the egg whites last.
2. Form burgers.
3. Heat a nonstick grill pan at medium temperature. Coat with cooking spray.
4. Add burgers to pan and cook 4 minutes on each side.
5. Serve with sautéed onions and whole-grain bread.

Turkey Meatballs
Serves 4

8 ounces ground turkey breast
1 tablespoon minced carrot
1 minced shallot
1 tablespoon reduced-fat Parmesan cheese
1 teaspoon Dijon mustard
1 teaspoon Worcestershire sauce
1 egg
1/2 cup whole-wheat pita bread crumbs
1 teaspoon dried basil
1 teaspoon dried oregano
Pinch of salt and pepper
Marinara Sauce (See recipe.)

Method:
1. In a large bowl, mix together all ingredients (except the Marinara Sauce).
2. Form mixture into 8 meatballs.
3. Heat a medium-sized skillet. Coat with cooking spray.
4. Place meatballs in skillet. Cover with Marinara Sauce and cook at medium-low temperature for 12 minutes. Stir gently occasionally.

Note: serve with Mushroom Gravy (see recipe).

ENTREES

Vegetarian Lasagna
Serves 4

8 whole-wheat lasagna noodles, cooked
1/2 cup sliced red pepper, steamed
1/2 cup small broccoli florets, steamed
1 cup spinach, cleaned and steamed
1/2 cup sliced onion, steamed
1/2 cup sliced carrot, steamed
1/2 cup julienne sun-dried tomatoes
1 teaspoon Italian seasoning
1 teaspoon crushed red pepper
2 cups Marinara Sauce (See Marinara Sauce recipe.)
16 ounces non-fat ricotta cheese
2 tablespoons reduced-fat Parmesan cheese
8 ounces part-skim milk mozzarella cheese

Method:
1. Preheat oven to 350° Fahrenheit.
2. In a Pyrex lasagna dish, layer bottom with 4 noodles, overlapping.
3. Top with the vegetables, tomatoes and 1 cup of the sauce.
4. Layer with 4 more noodles, overlapping.
5. Cover with remaining sauce and the cheese, adding the mozzarella cheese last.
6. Bake at 350° for 1 hour.

Baked Tomatoes
Serves 4

2 vine-ripened tomatoes cut into quarters
1 large firm yellow tomato, cut into quarters
1 tablespoon olive oil
Pinch of salt and pepper
2 egg whites
1/2 cup reduced-fat Parmesan cheese
1/4 cup whole-wheat pita crumbs

Method:
1. Preheat oven to 375° Fahrenheit.
2. In a large bowl, gently mix together the tomatoes, oil, salt and pepper.
3. Gently mix in egg whites.
4. In a separate bowl, mix together the Parmesan cheese and pita crumbs. Coat tomatoes with the mixture.
5. Place tomatoes on a nonstick baking sheet coated with cooking spray.
6. Bake at 375° for 10 minutes. Turn tomatoes once.

Bread Stuffing
Serves 4

2 cups egg bread
1 cup whole-wheat pita bread
4 cups water
1/2 cup saltines
1/2 cup minced onion
1/2 cup minced celery
1 tablespoon fresh Italian parsley, chopped
1 tablespoon fresh basil, chopped
2 tablespoons fresh dill, chopped
1 egg
Pinch of salt and pepper
1 tablespoon I Can't Believe It's Not Butter, melted

Method:
1. Preheat oven to 375° Fahrenheit.
2. In a bowl, soak egg bread and pita bread in 4 cups of water for 15 minutes.
3. Drain water from bowl and squeeze out remaining water from the bread until fairly dry.
4. Crumble saltines and mix into bread.
5. Mix in remaining ingredients.
6. Coat a 9-inch Pyrex baking dish with cooking spray.
7. Spoon mixture evenly into baking dish. Pour butter over the top.
8. Bake at 375° for 20 minutes.

French Green Beans Almondine
Serves 4

1 tablespoon olive oil
1 pound French green beans, ends cut
1 clove minced garlic
1/4 cup slivered almonds (toasted in 350° Fahrenheit oven for 5 minutes)
1 teaspoon fresh chopped thyme
Pinch of salt and pepper

Method:
1. Heat a medium skillet, add oil.
2. Add beans and garlic. Cook at medium-high temperature for 5 minutes, stirring frequently.
3. Add almonds, thyme, salt and pepper. Stir.

Herb-crusted Broccoli and Cauliflower
Serves 4

2 tablespoons olive oil
1 cup broccoli florets
1 cup cauliflower florets
1 teaspoon dried oregano
1 teaspoon Italian seasoning
2 tablespoons fresh chopped basil
1/2 teaspoon cayenne pepper
1 egg
1/2 cup whole-wheat pita bread crumbs
1/2 cup reduced-fat Parmesan cheese

Method:
1. Preheat oven to 375° Fahrenheit.
2. In a medium bowl, gently mix together the oil, broccoli and cauliflower.
3. Mix in the spices.
4. Gently fold in the egg.
5. In a separate bowl, coat the broccoli and cauliflower with the breadcrumbs and cheese.
6. Place coated broccoli and cauliflower on nonstick baking sheet.
7. Bake at 375° for 10 minutes.

SIDE DISHES

Roasted Potato Skin Wedges
Serves 2

1 baking potato, rinsed and scrubbed
  (Pat dry, cut into thin wedges with skin.)

2 teaspoons olive oil
1 teaspoon Italian seasoning
Pinch of salt and pepper
1/2 teaspoon paprika

Method:
1. Preheat oven to 375° Fahrenheit.
2. Mix potato wedges, oil and spices.
3. Place on nonstick baking sheet.
4. Bake at 375°, turning once, for 10 minutes.

Roasted Vegetable Medley
Serves 4

1/2 cup broccoli florets
1/2 cup cauliflower florets
1 cup asparagus spears
1/2 cup red pepper, large-diced
1/2 cup yellow pepper, large-diced
1/2 cup carrot slices
1/2 cup shitake mushroom halves
2 tablespoons olive oil
1 teaspoon Italian seasoning
1/2 teaspoon paprika
1/2 teaspoon oregano
Pinch of salt and pepper

Method:
1. Preheat oven to 375° Fahrenheit.
2. Place all ingredients in a large bowl and gently toss together, coating vegetables evenly.
3. Bake on nonstick baking sheet at 375° for 8 minutes.

Romanian Polenta with Fat-free Sour Cream
Serves 6

1 cup cornmeal
1 tablespoon matzo meal
1/2 teaspoon salt
2 tablespoons sugar or Splenda
3 egg whites
2 cups low-fat buttermilk
2 tablespoons non-fat sour cream

Topping:
1/2 cup of low-fat, pot-style cottage cheese
1/2 cup chopped scallions
4 tablespoons fresh chopped dill

Method:
1. Mix dry ingredients evenly.
2. Stir in buttermilk, egg whites and sour cream until smooth.
3. In a separate bowl, mix together cottage cheese, scallions and dill.
4. Pour batter into 8 x 8 Pyrex baking dish greased with cooking spray.
5. Spoon cottage cheese mixture evenly over the batter.
6. Bake for 45 minutes in a preheated oven at 350 degrees.
7. Remove from oven and let cool.
8. Cut into six squares and serve with a dollop of non-fat sour cream.

Saffron Pasta
Serves 2

1 tablespoon olive oil
1/4 cup julienne carrot
1/4 cup julienne peppers (3 colors)
1/4 cup sliced red onion
1/4 cup broccoli florets
1/4 cup sliced shitake mushrooms
1 cup cooked whole-wheat pasta spirals
1 tablespoon fresh basil, sliced
1 tablespoon reduced-fat Parmesan cheese

Cream sauce:
1/2 cup non-fat half and half
1 teaspoon saffron
1 teaspoon Dijon mustard
Pinch of salt and pepper

Method:
1. Simmer cream sauce ingredients in small saucepan until saffron releases color.
2. Heat a medium skillet, add olive oil.
3. Sauté vegetables until tender.
4. Mix in pasta.
5. Slowly add cream sauce until mix is slightly thick.
6. Top with basil and cheese.

Spinach with Garlic
Serves 4

1 tablespoon olive oil
1 pound fresh, cleaned spinach
1 teaspoon roasted garlic (minced)
2 tablespoons sun-dried tomato (julienne)

Method:
1. Heat a large pot to medium heat; add oil.
2. Cook all ingredients together at medium heat for 5 minutes or until spinach wilts. Stir frequently.

Vegetable Couscous
Serves 4

3 cups chicken broth, fat-free, low-sodium
1/4 cup diced celery
1/4 cup small broccoli florets
1/4 cup diced carrot
2 tablespoons minced onion
1/4 cup chopped sun-dried tomato
1/2 teaspoon curry
1/2 teaspoon cumin
Pinch of salt and pepper
2 cups couscous

Method:
1. Bring chicken broth, vegetables and tomato to a boil. Reduce heat, add curry, cumin, salt and pepper, and simmer for 5 minutes.
2. Bring broth back to a boil. Remove from stove.
3. Add couscous. Cover and set aside for 10 minutes.
4. Fluff with a fork and serve.

Suggestion: add raisins, dried cranberries and toasted pecans for a wonderful flavor.

Whipped Sweet Potatoes
Serves 4

4 medium sweet potatoes
1 tablespoon non-fat half and half

Method:
1. Preheat oven to 425° Fahrenheit.
2. Using a fork, pierce the sweet potatoes.
3. Wrap potatoes in aluminum foil.
4. Bake at 425° for 1 hour. Set potatoes aside to slightly cool, approximately 15 minutes.
5. Peel potatoes and place flesh into a food processor.
6. Cover. Pulsate potatoes while slowly adding half-and-half.
7. Place potato mixture into a pastry bag with a tip.
8. Form into swirls onto serving plates.

Wild-and Brown-Rice Pilaf
Serves 6

2 cups Lundberg wild-and-brown-rice blend
4 cups chicken broth, fat-free, low-sodium
1/4 cup chopped onion
1/4 cup diced carrot
1/4 cup dried red pepper
1/4 cup chopped mushrooms
1/2 cup diced sun-dried tomato
1 teaspoon Italian seasoning
Pinch of salt and pepper
1/4 cup chopped Italian parsley
1 tablespoon olive oil

Method:
1. Place all ingredients into a rice cooker (Hitachi) and press the On button. When rice pilaf is cooked, bell will ring.
2. Fluff rice with fork. Serve.

DESSERTS

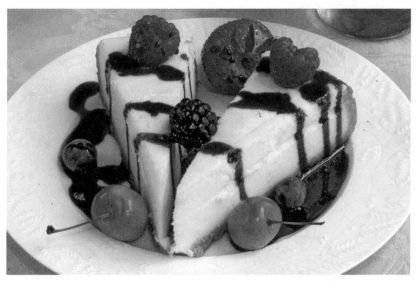

Low-fat, Sugar-free Cheesecake with Raspberry Coulis

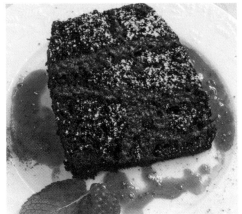

Double-layer Raspberry
Chocolate Cake

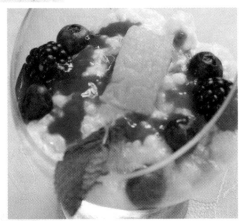

Light Custard with Berries

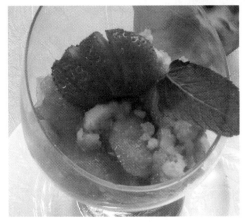

Peach Crumble

294

DESSERTS

Apple-cranberry Crumble
Serves 6

8 cups Granny Smith apples, peeled, cored and thinly sliced
1/4 cup Splenda sweetener
1 teaspoon apple pie spice
1 teaspoon cinnamon
1 teaspoon lemon juice
1/2 cup dried cranberries

Method:
In a large bowl, mix all ingredients together. Set apple mixture aside.

Crumble:
1/2 cup whole-wheat flour
1/2 cup unbleached flour
1 egg
2 tablespoons canola oil
1 tablespoon oats
1 teaspoon vanilla

Method:
1. Preheat oven to 375° Fahrenheit.
2. Mix together until smooth all of the crumble ingredients. Set aside.
3. Place the apple mixture into pie pan.
4. Evenly cover the apple mixture with the crumble.
5. Bake at 375° for 45 minutes.

DESSERTS

Blueberry Frozen Yogurt
Serves 4

2 cups non-fat, sugar-free vanilla yogurt
1 cup fresh blueberries

Method:
1. In a medium bowl, mix together the yogurt and the blueberries.
2. Scoop into parfait glasses and freeze for 1 hour or until semifrozen.

Double-layer Raspberry Chocolate Cake
Serves 8

1-1/2 cups whole-wheat flour
1-1/2 cups unbleached flour
2 cups Splenda sweetener
1/2 teaspoon salt
2 teaspoons baking soda
6 tablespoons powdered Dutch chocolate (cocoa)
1 cup canola oil
2 tablespoons white vinegar
2 teaspoons vanilla
3 cups water
4 tablespoons unsweetened raspberry preserves

Method:
1. Preheat oven to 375° Fahrenheit.
2. Sift together all of the dry ingredients into a large bowl.
3. Form three pockets in the dry mix.
4. In one pocket, pour the oil. In another pocket, pour the vinegar. In the third pocket, pour the vanilla. Cover with water and mix evenly.
5. Pour mixture into two 9-inch cake pans coated with an unflavored cooking spray.
6. Bake at 375° for 25 minutes
7. Let cakes cool for 30 minutes.
8. Release cakes from pans by turning upside down onto plates.
9. Spread raspberry preserves evenly over one cake. Place second cake on top to form the double-layer chocolate cake.

296

Light Custard with Berries
Serves 4

3 tablespoons tapioca custard mix
1 small container Egg Beaters
1/3 cup Splenda sweetener
2 cups non-fat half and half
3/4 cup skim milk
1 teaspoon vanilla extract
2 cups mixed berries (strawberries, raspberries,
    blueberries, blackberries)

Method:
1. Place all ingredients except berries into a large bowl and mix together.
2. Heat a medium saucepan. Add custard mixture and cook at medium temperature until it reaches a full boil. Stir frequently. Let cool for 15 minutes. Refrigerate approximately 1 hour to desired thickness.
3. Spoon custard into serving bowls and top with berry mix.

Suggestion: top with non-fat, sugar-free whipped topping.

Low-fat, Sugar-free Cheesecake
Serves 6

2 packages non-fat cream cheese
1 package 1/3 reduced-fat cream cheese
2 egg whites
1 egg
1/2 cup Splenda sweetener
1 teaspoon vanilla extract
1 ready-made reduced-fat piecrust

Method:
1. Preheat oven to 375° Fahrenheit.
2. Place all ingredients into a food processor. Cover.
3. Pulsate several times.
4. Blend until smooth (approximately 30 seconds).
5. Pour mixture into piecrust.
6. Reduce heat to 350° and bake for 1 hour or until toothpick inserted into center comes out clean.
7. Let cool for 15 minutes.
8. Refrigerate for 1 hour before serving.

Mixed Berry Crumble
Serves 6

1 cup blueberries
1 cup raspberries
1 cup blackberries
1 cup frozen cherries
1/2 cup red wine
1/4 cup Splenda sweetener
1 teaspoon cinnamon
1 teaspoon cornstarch
2 teaspoons water

Method:
1. In a large saucepan, add all ingredients except the cornstarch and water. Cook at medium temperature until mixture boils. Set fruit mixture aside.
2. Preheat oven to 375° Fahrenheit.
3. Mix cornstarch with the water.
4. Pour cornstarch into the center of the fruit mixture; stir until slightly thick. Set aside.

Crumble:
1/4 cup whole-wheat flour
1/4 cup unbleached flour
2 tablespoons canola oil
1 egg
1/4 cup Splenda sweetener
1 tablespoon oats

Method:
1. Mix crumble ingredients into smooth dough. Set aside.
2. Pour fruit mixture into a 9-inch Pyrex baking dish. Break the dough into crumble over the fruit mixture.
3. Bake at 375° for 45 minutes.

Peach Crumble
Serves 6

8 ripe peaches, peeled and sliced
1/4 cup Splenda sweetener
1 teaspoon cinnamon
2 tablespoons raisins
1/2 cup red wine

Method:
1. Heat all ingredients in a large saucepan until the wine is reduced. Set peach mixture aside.
2. Preheat oven to 375° Fahrenheit.

Crumble:
1/2 cup whole-wheat flour
1/2 cup unbleached flour
1 egg
1 teaspoon vanilla
1/4 cup Splenda sweetener
1 tablespoon oats
2 tablespoons canola oil
Mix all crumble ingredients together until smooth. Set aside.

Method:
1. Pour peach mixture into a 9-inch Pyrex pie pan (deep-dish).
2. Sprinkle with the crumble mixture, breaking crumble evenly over the top.
3. Bake at 375° for 45 minutes.

Raspberry Coulis
Serves 6

1 cup red wine
1 cinnamon stick
1 pint fresh raspberries (rinsed)
1/4 cup Splenda sweetener
2 tablespoons water

Method:
1. Heat a small saucepan; add red wine and cinnamon stick. Cook for 1 minute at medium temperature.
2. Add raspberries and Splenda. Lower temperature and simmer for 5 minutes. Set aside to cool.
3. Blend, adding water to achieve desired consistency. Note: coulis will thicken slightly when refrigerated.
4. Serve with low-fat cheesecake garnished with a strawberry and a mint sprig.

EPILOGUE

EPILOGUE

CREATING THE HEALTHIEST CAMPUS IN AMERICA

As I mentioned early on, my goal in writing this book has always been to share what I've learned over the years and to offer a perspective from my personal experience. Helping people live a healthier lifestyle is one of my passions, and as a result I'm working on several fronts to help get the word out about the benefits of living a healthy lifestyle.

The Seretean Wellness Center has been operating at Oklahoma State University since 1991. It was the first center on the campus of a large public institution to be dedicated solely to wellness. Today it operates almost 20 programs with an annual budget of $1.5 million. Serving students, faculty and the community, the Seretean Wellness Center offers everything from wellness education classes to risk assessments and annual screenings. It provides nutrition counseling as well as cooking demonstrations. The fitness center is one of the best on any university campus.

All along, our goal has been to increase awareness of the need for wellness and to encourage students, faculty and community members to live healthier lifestyles. But there's also another goal – one that might be harder to reach.

Working with the team at the Seretean Wellness Center and with the support of the administration at Oklahoma State, I'm hoping to have the university recognized as the healthiest institution of higher education in America. When we complete this goal, we will be, in essence, closing the circle we opened before the building's first brick was laid.

When we started the center, we focused on making sure wellness information on everything from stress, nutrition and exercise to the dangers of tobacco and alcohol was made available to the university community and to the people of Stillwater, who participate in programs at the center. We've come a long way in this endeavor, with the staff increasing from six to more than 40. I'm certain the message is getting out and the programs are proving to be successful.

EPILOGUE: CREATING THE HEALTHIEST CAMPUS IN AMERICA

We've seen some positive signs Oklahoma State is on the way to becoming America's healthiest campus. Already, class absenteeism has been reduced and we know that knowledge about wellness has been increasing. Almost all of the university's schools have a class on wellness designed for incoming freshmen, and as many as 50 percent of the students do take these classes. Students now are asking for increased amounts of healthy food in the cafeteria and are also taking advantage of the free blood screenings the university offers.

The student population at OSU, and just about any other university, is one that's transient, and it's difficult to follow success for long periods of time. But there are 2,000 to 3,000 members of the faculty and staff at Oklahoma State who are there for long periods of time and have become the focus of our efforts. As part of the program at the Seretean Wellness Center, we've established a health clinic for employees and their dependents. We also offer physical exams and, of course, make the facilities and courses available to the faculty and staff.

We've seen an increase in the number of faculty and staff members focusing on wellness, including the university president, Dr. David Schmidly, who now makes it a point to exercise on a regular basis. Without his active leadership, we would not have enjoyed the success we've achieved to date. The success of any wellness program depends on the commitment of the person in charge.

Another goal is to have Stillwater recognized as the healthiest city in the nation. The city has a big influence on the university and the university has a big impact on the city. Both must work together in order to be successful. We have met with city officials, from the mayor on down, and have helped the city set up a health committee. We have also met with local restaurants and gyms to help get the word out about wellness, and we're hoping to get grant money so the city can hire an epidemiologist to track its progress.

Why are we going through all this effort? Well, obviously the university will benefit if it can boast of having the healthiest campus in the country and it will also benefit from being located in the healthiest city in the nation. More out-of-state students will be drawn to the campus, and parents will feel good about sending their children off to a school where long-term health is emphasized.

EPILOGUE: CREATING THE HEALTHIEST CAMPUS IN AMERICA

But the most important reason for wanting to create the healthiest campus in the country and for wanting to create the healthiest city in America goes back to the very first pages of this book.

My goal for the last 25 years has been to share the information I've learned in the hope it will help people live longer and healthier lives. Wellness, as I've mentioned, is a lifelong process of striving for a healthy balance in physical and mental health. If we can introduce people to it earlier in their lives, they might indeed make it a way of life. If both OSU and Stillwater are successful in achieving these goals, what terrific role models they'll become for universities and cities all over the country.

It's never too late to start. I hope as you've read this book, you've been able to find reasons to make a change in your life and focus on a healthier lifestyle. If this book helps just one person move toward a healthier lifestyle, then the effort that has gone into it will have been worthwhile.

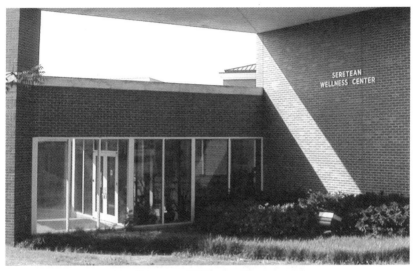

Seretean Wellness Center
Oklahoma State University
Stillwater, Oklahoma

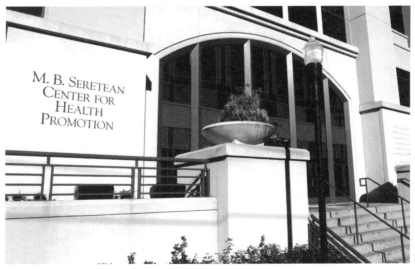

M.B. Seretean Center for Health Promotion
Emory University
Atlanta, Georgia

ABOUT THE AUTHOR

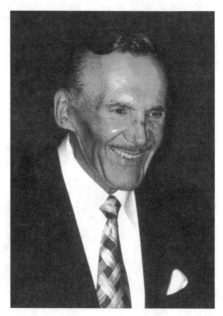

M.B. "Bud" Seretean

A successful entrepreneur, philanthropist and strong supporter of healthy living, M.B. "Bud" Seretean has spent the past 25 years learning about and promoting wellness and living a lifestyle that includes eating well, exercising regularly and managing stress.

A native New Yorker who sold popcorn at Yankee Stadium, Seretean grew up in his family's grocery store, knowing nothing of the hazards associated with high-fat foods. After four years in the service during World War II serving as a field artillery officer in the Mediterranean theater, Seretean graduated from Oklahoma State University with a degree in marketing and later earned a master's degree from New York University.

Starting his career as an assistant buyer of floor coverings for a department store, Seretean in 1956 cofounded Coronet Industries, a carpet manufacturing business that quickly grew to $400 million in annual sales and more than 4,000 employees. The company was sold to RCA Corp. in 1971 and Seretean's lifelong interest in sports led him to become president and general manager of the Atlanta Hawks basketball team during the 1970s.

It was during a 1979 visit to the Pritikin Longevity Center in Pennsylvania that Seretean made a commitment to living a healthy lifestyle and to promoting that lifestyle so others could share in its benefits. He is the driving force behind the Seretean Wellness Center at Oklahoma State University, the first center of its kind on a college campus, and also provided funding for the Seretean Health Promotion Center at Emory University in Atlanta. His generosity led to the building of the Seretean Center for the Performing Arts, also on the campus of Oklahoma State, and to numerous scholarships. Seretean also supports scientific research promoting a healthy lifestyle.

In 1999, he received an honorary doctorate on the 50th anniversary of his graduation from Oklahoma State University in recognition of his professional accomplishments and his philanthropic activities. He was awarded the 10th honorary doctorate from the university, with previous recipients including Henry Kissinger and President George H.W. Bush.

Today Mr. Seretean lives in Boca Raton, Florida, where he continues to lead a healthy lifestyle. He remains active in the promotion of wellness at Oklahoma State University and speaks to groups throughout the country about healthy living.

READING/SOURCES LIST
&
SERVICES FOR SENIORS

READING/SOURCES LIST

Books

Ageless, Take Control of Your Age and Stay Youthful for Life by Edward L. Schneider, M.D., and Elizabeth Miles. (Rodale Press Inc., distributed to the book trade by St. Martin's Press, 2003)

Age Wave, The Challenges and Opportunities of an Aging America by Ken Dychtwald, Ph.D. and Joe Flower. (J. P. Tarcher, Inc., distributed by St. Martin's Press, 1989)

American Dietetic Association Complete Food and Nutrition Guide, 2nd edition by Roberta Larson Duyff. (John Wiley & Sons, Inc., 2002)

The American Vegetarian Cookbook: From the Fit for Life Kitchen by Marilyn Diamond. (Warner Books, 1990)

Dr. Dean Ornish's Program for Reversing Heart Disease: the only system scientifically proven to reverse heart disease without drugs or surgery by Dean Ornish M.D. (Random House, Inc., 1990)

Drug Interaction Facts: 2004, edited by David S. Tatro. (Facts and Comparisons Publishing Group, 2004)

Eat, Drink and Be Healthy: The Harvard Medical School Guide to Healthy Eating by Walter C. Willett, M.D. (Simon and Schuster, 2001)

Eat More and Weigh Less: Dr. Dean Ornish's Life Choice Program for Losing Weight Safely While Eating Abundantly by Dean Ornish, M.D. (HarperCollins, 1993; revised and updated 2001)

The New York Times Guide to Alternative Health: a consumer reference by Jane E. Brody, Denise Grady and the reporters of The New York Times. (Times Books, Henry Holt and Company, 2001)

READING/SOURCES LIST

The Nutrition Bible, A Comprehensive, No-Nonsense Guide to Foods, Nutrients, Additives, Preservatives, Pollutants, and Everything Else We Eat and Drink by Jean Anderson and Barbara Deskins. (Morrow, 1995)

Picture Perfect Weight Loss: The Visual Program for Permanent Weight Loss by Dr. Howard M. Shapiro. (Rodale, Inc.; distributed to the book trade by St. Martin's Press, 2000)

The Pritikin Permanent Weight-Loss Manual by Nathan Pritikin. (Grosset & Dunlap, 1981)

The Pritikin Program for Diet and Exercise by Nathan Pritikin with Patrick M. McGrady, Jr. (Grosset & Dunlap, 1979)

Too Busy to Count the Years by Suzanne Snyder Jacobson. (Andrews McMeel Publishing, 2001)

The Benefits and Risks of Vitamins and Minerals: What You Need to Know, a Special Health Report from Harvard Medical School, Harvard Health Publications.

Articles

"The ABCs of Diabetes" by Christine Gorman, *TIME magazine*, April 14, 2003

"Carbohydrates Without Fear" *Consumer Reports on Health,* October 2003

"Cereal Trends: Not Your Mother's Rice Krispies" by Bonnie Liebman and Jane Hurley, *Nutrition Action HealthLetter,* November 2003

"Cholesterol: How Low Should You Go?" *Consumer Reports on Health,* March 2004

"Dining Out Tips" *Pritikin Perspective,* September/October 1998

READING/SOURCES LIST

"Female and Fit for Life" *Nutrition Action HealthLetter*, May 2004

"Happier and Healthier" *Consumer Reports on Health*, March 2004

"Health for Life: Beyond the Fads: What Science Tells Us About Food and Health" special section, *Newsweek*, January 20, 2003

"How to Stay Healthy in 2002" *TIME magazine, Medicine and Prevention Issue*, January 28, 2002

"How Accurate Are Food Claims?" *Consumer Reports on Health*, October 2002

"Leisure Time Exercises" *Harvard Men's Health Watch*, May 2004

"Nutrition for Seniors: Options and Opportunities" *Harvard Men's Health Watch*, June 2004

"Pressure Points: 7 Facts About Hypertension You Can't Afford to Ignore" *Nutrition Action HealthLetter*, April 2004

"Putting New Wrinkles on Prunes' Health Benefits" by Brandy Jones, reprinted by permission from *The DailyOklahoman*. Based on "The Effects of Prunes on Bone in Ovarian Hormone Deficiency," a laboratory study on rats conducted by Dr. Bahram Arjmandi, Dr. Barbara Stoecker, Dr. Edralin Lucas, Oklahoma State University, College of Human Environmental Sciences. Funded by the California Prune Board, 1999

"Risk Factors from Homocysteine: from Ask the Experts: Tips from the Registered Dieticians, Exercise Physiologists and Scientists at the Prikikin Longevity Center," *Pritikin Perspective*, January 1998

"Stronger Bones Without the Hype" *Consumer Reports on Health*, May 2004

READING/SOURCES LIST

"Weighing the Diet Books" *Nutrition Action HealthLetter*, January/February 2004

"Why Are We So Fat?" by Cathy Newman, *National Geographic*, August 2004

Online

"Arthritis Advice," National Institute on Aging, January 2002
www.niapublications.org/engagepages/arthritis.asp

"Diet Wars," FRONTLINE, Public Broadcasting System, 2004. For text of television program or to view it online:
www.pbs.org/wgbh/pages/frontline/shows/diet

"Dietary Fiber Fights High Blood Pressure," ABC News, HealthDay News, Inc., March 4, 2005; www.healthday.com

"Drug Interaction Facts," Facts & Comparisons Publishing Group, www.drugfacts.com

"Fat Distribution Key to Health Risk," updated March, 2005, www.preventdisease.com

"High Fiber," McKinley Health Center, University of Indiana at Urbana-Champagne, www.mckinley.uiuc.edu

"Omega-3 Fatty Acids," *Whole Health MD*, Sterling, Virginia, www.wholehealthmd.com

Ornish, Dr. Dean at PMRI (Preventative Medicine Research Institute), www.ornish.com

"Prostate Cancer and Diet: Animal Fat (Bad) and Soy (Good) May Cause 10-fold Difference in U.S. vs. Japan," *PR NewsWire*, October 21, 2004, http://www.usrf.org/japanese-american_cap/jpam.pdf

READING/SOURCES LIST

"Protecting Women's Hearts Gets Personal: New Guidelines Issued for Preventing Heart Disease and Stroke in Women," by Jennifer Warner, *Web MD Health*, February 20, 2004, www.mywebmd.com

"Questions and Answers About Trans Fat Nutrition Labeling," U.S. Food and Drug Administration, Center for Food Safety and Applied Nutrition, July 2003, updated June 2004, www.cfsan.fda.gov/~dms/qatrans2.html

"Soy Foods May Combat Prostate Cancer," *PSA Rising*, from a presentation by Dr. Mark Messina, October 1999, Annual Meeting of the American College of Nutrition, Washington, D.C., www.psa-rising.com

"'Superfoods' Everyone Needs," by Gina Shaw, *WebMD Health*, Feb. 10, 2004; copyright WebMD, Inc., www.mywebmd.com

SERVICES FOR SENIORS

AARP (American Association for Retired Persons)
Non-profit, nonpartisan organization for people age 50 and over that provides a wide range of benefits, products and services for its members.

> **General Information**
> 601 E. Street NW
> Washington, DC 20049
> 888-OUR-AARP (888-687-2277) for information.
> To speak to a representative, say the word "representative"
> Fax: 202-434-6474, 202-434-7599
> www.aarp.org

AARP Foundation – Featured Employers Program
A listing of employers who hire mature workers.
www.aarp.org/money/careers/findingajob/featuredemployers/

AARP Grandparent Information Center
Provides assistance for grandparents, including those raising grandchildren, as well as information regarding support groups and agencies
www.aarp.org/life/grandparents

Alzheimer's Disease Education and Referral Center (ADEAR)
P.O. Box 8250
Silver Spring, MD 20907-8250
800-438-4380
Fax: 301-495-3334
www.alzheimers.org

America's Seniors/Today's Seniors Network
Newsletter for seniors via e-mail with news on issues of concern to older Americans and other subjects, such as entertainment.
www.todaysseniorssnetwork.com

American Cancer Society
1599 Clifton Rd NE
Atlanta GA 30329
800-ACS-2345 (800-227-2345)
www.cancer.org

American Council of the Blind
1155 15th Street NW, Suite 1004
Washington, DC 20005
800-424-8666
Fax: 202-467-5085
www.acb.org

American Health Assistance Foundation
22512 Gateway Center Drive
Clarksburg, MD 20871
800-437-AHAF (2423)
Fax: 301-258-9454
www.ahaf.org

American Heart Association
7272 Greenville Avenue
Dallas, TX 75231
800-AHA-USA1 (800-242-8721)
www.americanheart.org

SERVICES FOR SENIORS

American Lung Association
61 Broadway, 6th Floor
New York, NY 10006
800-Lung-USA (to connect to your local organization)
www.lungusa.org

Arthritis Foundation
P.O. Box 7669
Atlanta, GA 30357-0669
800-568-4045
www.arthritis.org

Association of Jewish Family and Children's Agencies
620 Cranbury Road, Suite 102
East Brunswick, NJ 08816
800-634-7346
Fax: 732-432-7127
www.ajfca.org

Catholic Charities USA
1731 King Street
Alexandria, VA 22314
Phone: 703-549-1390
Fax: 703-549-1656
www.catholiccharitiesusa.org
www.catholiccharitiesinfo.org/contact/index.cfm (for local information)

Experience Works, Inc.
National non-profit organization that works to improve economic and social conditions of older Americans and their families by providing essential services and promoting employment and training.
2200 Clarendon Blvd., Suite 1000
Arlington, VA 22201
866-EXP-WRKS (866-397-9757)
Fax: 703-522-0141
www.experienceworks.org

Family Caregiver Alliance
180 Montgomery St., Suite 1100
San Francisco, CA 94104
800-445-8106
Fax: 415-434-3508
info@caregiver.org
www.caregiver.org

Grandparents Raising Grandchildren
Provides information on state and local resources.
www.firstgov.gov/Topics/Grandparents

Institute for the Study of Aging
1414 Avenue of the Americas
Suite 1502
New York, NY 10019
212-935-2402
Fax: 212-935-2408
www.aging-institute.org

Meals on Wheels

Find local Meals on Wheels and other meal delivery and congregate meal services for senior citizens. Also provides links to other sources to assist seniors, including senior homecare, housing and in-home assisted living.
www.mealcall.org

Medicare

Centers for Medicare & Medicaid Services
7500 Security Boulevard
Baltimore MD 21244-1850
800-MEDICARE (800-633-4227)
www.medicare.gov

Medicare Hotline

Assistance with Medicare problems or questions, concerning insurance, counseling and assistance programs and local agencies.
Families USA/Shortchanged,
1201 New York Ave., Suite 1100
Washington, DC 20005
800-MEDICARE (800-633-4227)
www.familiesusa.org

NIA (National Institute on Aging)

Senior-friendly website from the National Institutes of Health and National Library of Medicine. Features popular health topics for older adults, large type and "talking" function that reads the text out loud.
31 Center Dr., MSC 2292
Building 31, Room 5C27
Bethesda, MD 20892
www.nia.nih.gov

National Association for Visually Handicapped
Non-profit association providing assistance to those with partial vision. Low vision services, visual aids and training.
22 West 21st Street, 6th Floor
New York, NY 10010
212- 889-3141
Fax: 212- 727-2931
www.navh.org

The National Blueprint: Increasing Physical Activity Among Adults Age 50 and Older
Provides information about organizations and agencies promoting physical activity for seniors.
www.agingblueprint.org

National Family Caregivers Association
10400 Connecticut Avenue, Suite 500
Kensington, MD 20895-3944
800-896-3650
Fax: 301-942-2302
www.nfcacares.org

National Federation of the Blind
Provides necessary information for the blind.
1800 Johnson St.
Baltimore, MD 21230
410-659-9314
Fax: 410-685-5653
www.nfb.org

National Osteoporosis Foundation
1232 22nd Street, NW
Washington, DC 20037-1292
202 223-2226
Fax: 202 223-2237
www.nof.org
Support Groups: finding or starting osteoporosis support groups
www.nof.org/patientinfo/support_groups.htm

National Respite Network and Resource Center
800 Eastowne Drive, Suite 105
Chapel Hill, NC 27514
919-490-5577
Fax: 919-490-4905
www.archrespite.org

Post - polio Support
For support group in your area, e-mail queries to:
G.I.N.I._International_gini_intl@msn.com

SHHH (Self-Help for Hard of Hearing People)
Educates people with hearing losses to help themselves enjoy their life
to the fullest.
7910 Woodmont Ave, Suite 1200
Bethesda, Maryland 20814
301-657-2248
Fax: 301-913-9413
www.shhh.org

SERVICES FOR SENIORS

Senior Artesians Online Marketplace
E-commerce website that provides senior artisans and crafters a nationwide marketplace for their handcrafted goods
Geezer.com Customer Service Center
2700 Pecan Street, #525
Pflugerville, TX 78660
877-803-1468
www.geezer.com to apply to place your work online, click "About Us"

Senior Corps Network
Network of national service programs that provide senior Americans the opportunity to apply their life experiences to meeting community needs.
Foster Grandparent Program
Senior Companion Program
RSVP (Retired and Senior Volunteer Program)
800-424-8867
www.seniorcorps.org

Senior Mentors Program
This is a yearlong program, 20-40 hours per week.
Sponsored by FIRST (For Inspiration and Recognition of Science and Technology), which motivates young people to pursue opportunities in science, technologies and engineering.
200 Bedford St.
Manchester, NH 03101
603-666-3906
Fax: 603-666-3907
www.usfirst.org/about/sr_mentors
www.usfirst.org

SERVICES FOR SENIORS

U.S.A. Harvest
Feeding the hungry from coast to coast.
800-USA.4FOOD
800-872-4366
www.usaharvest.com

World Animal Net
Worldwide database for local agencies, adoption, rescue, care and
assistance for all kinds of animals.
19 Chestnut Square
Boston, MA 02130
617-524-3670
Fax: 360-364-7347
www.worldanimalnet.org

YMCA
A variety of programs, classes and services for people of all ages,
including seniors. Local branch and program information at
www.ymca.net

YWCA USA
Programs and activities for girls and women and for seniors of both
sexes.
1015 18th Street, NW, Suite 1100
Washington, DC 20036
202-467-0801
Fax: 202-467-0802
www.ywca.org

INDEX

INDEX

INDEX

INDEX